LEWY BODY & PARKINSONISM DEMENTIAS

A Guide for Doctors, Nurses, Patients, Families, Students, & Caregivers

JERRY BELLER HEALTH RESEARCH INSTITUTE

DEDICATION

To people living with Dementia and their loved ones.

CONTENTS

ACKNOWLEDGMENTS

Thanks to the American Academy of Neurology, Atlanta Center for Medical Research, Alzheimer's Association, Alzheimer's Disease Center, Alzheimer's Disease Center of Northwestern University, Alzheimer's Foundation of America, American Academy of Neurology, Association for Frontotemporal Degeneration, Australia Neurological Research, CDC, Department of Health and Human Services, Duke University Medical Center, Emory Hospital, Harvard Medical School, Johns Hopkins Medicine, Mayo Clinic, National Aphasia Association, National Institute of Neurological Disorders and Strokes, National Library of Medicine, National Institute on Aging, National Institutes of Health, Prince of Wales Medical Research Institute, *PubMed*, Stanford Library School of Medicine, Stanford Medicine, UCSF Department of Neurology, UCSF Memory and Aging Center, University of Cambridge Neurology Unit, World Health Organization (WHO), *Journal of American Medical Association* (JAMA), and several other organizations that provided information used for this book. Thanks to everybody who assisted this book in a variety of important ways, and everybody at Beller Health Research Institute. To my editor, John Briggs, who helps me improve every book. To all sources and for the photos. Most of all, thanks to my wife, Nicola Beller

FOREWORD

Before diving into the book's subject matter, let's discuss two related Dementia series:

- *2020 Dementia Overview* series
- *2020 Dementia Types, Symptoms, Stages, & Risk Factors* series

2020 Dementia Overview series is an extension of the medical groundbreaking *19 Dementia Types, Symptoms, Stages, & Risk Factors* series, the first covering all primary dementia types.

After spending decades building an audience in other genres, including nutrition, circumstances turned the world upside down. Doctors diagnosed my mother with Alzheimer's. The same doctors soon diagnosed my father with cancer. A few months later, my father's favorite brother and my closest uncle died.

Three consecutive hard blows blew the world beyond recognition.

Tough and decent as they come, dad insisted on taking care of my mother while fighting brain cancer. My brothers and sister-in-law did their share, but Dad cared for my mother for a long time while they worked. Dad proved what a remarkable and great man he was down the stretch but finally succumbed to brain cancer.

My brothers and sister-in-law did their best to take care of mom, but it came at a price. Caregiving for a dementia patient is an indescribable horror I would not wish on my worst enemy.

You must watch somebody you love wilt away, little by little until dementia wipes away huge chunks of their personality.

Living away, my wife and I visited when possible. We saw how mom deteriorated, but also the effect caregiving had on my father and brothers. It was like watching a train wreck over and over, each time getting worse and helpless to prevent it.

Watching Alzheimer's takedown, my strong-willed mother and others bruised my soul. My writing shifted initially to learn about Alzheimer's, but the more learned, the more I cringed.

The cold hard facts rendered me speechless. Over 5.8 million Americans, and 44 million people worldwide, suffer Alzheimer's. No cure. Just a devastating and expensive slow march towards an agonizing end.

Not content to kill, Alzheimer's tortured Mom for years before killing her. It robbed her memory and damaged her brain, where she repeated herself in a continuous loop, each time thinking she was saying it the first time. As the disease advanced, the neurological disorder destroyed her mind and body.

Seeing dementia take down that tough old bird rattled me. While I could not bring back my mother, I dedicate my life to researching and writing about dementia 8-12 hours per day, six or seven days per week.

I tackled Alzheimer's to learn everything I could about the brute and determine how I and others might prevent it and other noncommunicable diseases. Having written on nutrition and advocated health in Washington, I already had a clue but determined to figure out how to prevent Alzheimer's. But I needed to know more, much more, about this terrorizing neurological disorder.

I learned Alzheimer's was just one of over one-hundred neurological disorders causing dementia. When I searched for a book covering the primary dementias, none existed. Instead, I turned to individual books and again found no books written on several of the most frequent dementias.

In what on the one hand seems like yesterday and the other a lifetime ago, I set out several years ago to write a dementia book covering the 15 most prevalent dementia types. The first to do that, I next wrote books covering each of the 15 most prevalent dementias.

In 2020, I expanded the book covering 15 dementias to 19 dementia types. I also released books on each of the 19 dementias. While proud of these medical firsts, I do not take myself too seriously.

As one of the dozens of scientists, neurologists, researchers, and writers who devote their lives to fighting the war against dementia, I remain humble. I appreciate the individual and combined accomplishments of everybody else in the field.

Nor should any of us get cocky knowing we're losing the war. If we win the war during my lifetime, I will celebrate with hundreds of people worldwide who helped defeat the great beast of our day.

My two-book series break medical ground, and I consider major achievements but remain two among hundreds of significant contributions to the dementia field by people around the globe.

The series provides patients and loved ones a great resource for dementias not covered as extensive as Alzheimer's and the more prevalent types.

By covering the 19 most prevalent dementias, doctors, nurses, and medical professionals benefit from a series covering neurological disorders causing 99% of dementia. The series helps primary care physicians, providers, and nurses who struggle to diagnose dementias with overlapping symptoms.

The series is an organic, evolving work, and each book receives major annual updates. As science uncovers information, we add important data in new editions. We also polish each edition.

We describe the writing goal in three ways:

1. Simplify the language and make it easier for nonscientists to comprehend.
2. Honor the science and facts.
3. Document science and include citations for doctors,

nurses, medical researchers, students, and patients.

Our goal is to provide invaluable medical information for professionals, patients, loved ones, and caregivers.

I do not reinvent the wheel but accumulate the best research and teach our readers a better understanding of Alzheimer's and the other 18 primary dementia types.

Among the worst news is one of our loved ones has dementia. A killer disease with no cure frightens the bravest souls.

This medical condition destroys, not just the inflicted, but their loved ones. Besides the patient, nobody suffers more than voluntary caregivers. Watching a mother, father, brother, sister, wife, or husband suffering dementia brutalizes the soul.

I study dementia year around to write and release annual updates to honor people—including my mother—taken by Alzheimer's or one of the other primary dementias.

Modest book royalties are the only compensation, as I accept no money from corporations to promote their product. Nor do I have an ax to grind with anybody in the medical profession.

Having written 100 plus books over four decades, I am thankful to readers for collectively providing me a decent income. However, now in my sixties, I care little about riches and fame.

Who is the reading audience?

The audience falls into five categories.

Those Diagnosed with Dementia

If doctors diagnose you with dementia, my heart goes out to you. You're in for a long battle. Do yourself a favor and focus on slowing the disease and extending the quality of life. One word of caution, the books in this series speak to not only patients, but also families, doctors, students, nurses, and caregivers. Many of those diagnosed with dementia appreciate and benefit from the books, but some find some of the material too disturbing. I intend to write books exclusively for patients but must finish the work related to this series first. While there is not anything too shocking, I wrote the material for a wide audience, meaning I am not always speaking to patients specifically. I promise to personalize an edition for patients and loved ones after finishing this series. By shining a light on all 19 primary dementia types, I hope to help the medical community better distinguish and diagnose neurological disorders.

Loved Ones of Those Diagnosed

If doctors diagnose a loved one with dementia, he or she needs you more than ever. Depending on the type, dementia causes behavioral problems, memory issues, motor decline, and other psychological and physical disorders. The learning curve is steep and changes as one moves from one stage to the next. As with those with dementia, I warn families these books provide a technical overview, and the emphasis is not always on the emotional aspect. If you want to learn about dementias, this series is a great option. If you're looking more for emotional support, there are more appropriate books. I also plan to write a book specifically for families once fulfilling responsibilities for this series.

Medical Professionals

If you are a medical professional interested in studying the dementias, the series covers the dementias responsible for 99% of dementia. While neurologists probably already know the 19 primary dementias, the books provide a quick overview and reference for primary care physicians, nurses, other medical professionals, and students. I also include citations so you can continue your investigation beyond the book's scope.

Volunteer & Professional Caregivers

If you are a dementia caregiver, you are also in for a long, difficult march. Dementia patients demand 24/7 care in later stages, requiring help to go to the bathroom, bathing, and other basic daily functions. While this series is not written solely for caregiving, caregivers benefit by gaining a better understanding of each dementia, their symptoms, and progression.

Anybody Wanting to Learn About A Disease That Strikes 1 Of 6 Americans, And 1 Of 3 Seniors

The series benefits anybody who wants to gain an intermediate understanding of the 19 dementias.

Series' First Lesson

Doctors, like teachers, are part of a sacred profession. **Nothing I say or write replaces your need for a competent doctor!** Nor does any criticism of the profession diminish my respect and admiration for the best.

I detest the worst teachers who fail students and society but love and respect the best. Society would crumble without the most devoted and competent teachers.

Similar, I abhor incompetent, greedy doctors who fail patients and society, but love and respect the best.

The profession must weed out incompetent, uncaring, corrupt doctors, and medical personnel. Every profession has a percentage of bad apples, but within the medical profession, they are cancerous!

Nothing good I write about the medical profession includes incompetent, uncaring doctors, researchers, nurses, etc. And nothing bad I write targets the best.

The series criticizes the profession when deserved, but the first lesson in this series: **Find a competent doctor!** If you have one, count your blessings. If not, find one.

Just as one can learn outside the classroom, we live in a blessed age where medical information is available for anybody on the internet. Such information serves us well, but do not—for a minute-think it replaces the need for a competent, devoted doctor.

The Wrong Doctors

Let me begin this section by saying I love and respect quality doctors, nurses, researchers, and medical professionals from the bottom of my heart and the fullness of my mind.

However, this section is not about what's right in the medical profession.

Glorified idiots, bad doctors are dangerous parasites who dishonor a noble profession. Smart enough to finish medical school, but greedy or flawed beyond redemption, they are like priests working for the devil. Among the worse members of society are doctors motivated by greed or limited by incompetence. Walking parasites!

The Wrong Doctors + Big Pharm + Big Insurance + Big Hospital = Expensive & Inadequate Health Care

Over the past few decades, Big pharmaceuticals, Big Insurance, and their political puppets appointed doctors sanctioned drug dealers. Entrusting the worse doctors with such powers produces little or no better results than assigning the task to a thug on the worst corner in America.

The worst doctors who hand out drugs like candy serve nobody's purpose but their own and Big Pharm.

Not an indictment of the entire profession, but unfortunately, Big Insurance dictates the typical office visit includes a quick examination and one or more prescriptions. The approach is not based on good science and runs counter to everything science teaches us.

JERRY BELLER HEALTH RESEARCH INSTITUTE

What About Some Tough Love?

The one thing people today do not want is what we often need most, tough love. People want everything sugarcoated and easy.

The problem is most of the time; life is neither sweet nor easy.

What patients need much of the time is not an alleged "magic pill," but instead tough love. Doctors must learn nutrition and teach patients to eat healthier, exercise more, and get 7-8 hours of sleep per night. Like it or not, this is part of modern medicine. Showing up and passing out pills all day is not preventing Alzheimer's and other dementias, nor curing them.

Medical professionals must lead by example and embrace the science of nutrition, exercise, and sleep. If a healthy diet and exercise are the two cornerstones to health, the third is sleep.

The average person needs few or no drugs if they practice healthy habits.

Any doctor who does not vigorously advocate a balanced whole food diet, exercise most days of the week, and 7-8 hours' sleep per night neglects their duty and

Instead, too many doctors ignore the three cornerstones of health and are content to write their patients unnecessary and potentially dangerous prescriptions for the rest of their lives. 100% emphasis on treating symptoms with drugs, which often require more drugs to counter the side effects, is producing disastrous results. To be the best doctor, one must also emphasize prevention.

Failed Drug Trials

None of the drug trials have produced even one drug that cures Alzheimer's and other dementias. While science has failed to produce any effective dementia drugs, scientific studies prove we can do much by practicing healthy habits to slow or reduce our dementia risk.

The Medical Profession Must Think Outside The Box

The hopeless circle of failed drug trials demands we think outside the box or, as neurologist David Perlmutter advocates, expand the box. He and other neurologists deserve credit for recognizing medicine is failing the dementia war and rocking the boat of conventional wisdom. I must not agree with every point "maverick" neurologists like David Perlmutter, Dale Bredesen, and Deepak Chopra make to respect them for turning conventional wisdom on its head.

Conventional wisdom is losing the Alzheimer's and dementia war!

Not Anti-doctors or Anti-drugs

I am not anti-doctors or anti-drugs and do not understand those who insist neither are needed. I revere competent doctors who practice and advocate the three cornerstones of health. I also recognize the polio vaccine and many other drugs as nothing short of miraculous.

But, my love for what is right about the medical profession will not silence me about what is wrong. And, pretending drugs are the answer to defeating Alzheimer's or dementia is a colossal failure.

You cannot "**do no harm**" and write prescription drugs at the volume of the average doctor.

Choose A Doctor with The Same Care As You Do A Spouse

Find a competent, dedicated, caring, experienced, informed, ethical doctor who listens and respects your opinion, and writes prescriptions as a LAST RESORT.

Without the right doctor, you are at the mercy of a profit-oriented health system that seldom puts the patient's interests first, second, or third.

Nothing I say or write in these books or elsewhere means you should not see a doctor, stop taking your medication, or otherwise undermine the medical profession's ability to diagnose and treat any medical symptoms you might experience.

Find a good doctor you trust with your life and ask him or her pointed questions concerning your health and any treatment they recommend.

Outside the Bubble

I challenge the medical profession where necessary, just as I criticize Congress and the United States government for their mistakes or shortcomings. My brief career as a Congressional staffer taught me how difficult it is to maintain one's focus inside the bubble.

Seeing the big picture is no less challenging inside the medical bubble motivated by profit.

Profiteers fund too many studies to promote their product or discredit somebody else's. Blatant self-interests taint studies and confuse the public. Such contradictory studies confuse and make it impossible for the average person to understand which studies to believe.

I respect ethical, competent, dedicated, and hardworking nurses, doctors, and other medical personnel. As much as I criticize what is wrong within the profession, I cannot praise the majority of medical professionals often enough. Getting quality medical care when we need it is one of life's greatest blessings.

Nor do I object to medical-related businesses making a reasonable profit in return for needed medical supplies and services.

Nor should any competent and ethical medical professionals object to anybody challenging medical incompetence and profiteers.

Trust Thy Doctor

The right doctor does not discriminate between physical and mental diseases, so hold back nothing if you or a loved one exhibits symptoms.

If you lack the right doctor, find the right one. Outside you and the daily habits you establish, nobody is more important than your doctor for your health. You must be able to tell him or her medical information you might be reluctant to tell your closest confidant in life.

Remember, doctors too often misdiagnose dementia. Once the symptoms of these deadly dementias set in, you need to see your doctor, provide them with all the information about your problem, and help the specialists reach the correct diagnosis.

Because no tests exist for most dementias, doctors order tests and go through a process of elimination until reaching a diagnosis based on the symptoms you report. The more information you provide, the better the chance of a quick and accurate diagnosis.

Adopt healthy lifestyle choices to prevent dementia when possible, but the next best option is to diagnose it early, to confront it head-on, and take steps to slow the disease. Once dementia hits, it's often possible to postpone the advanced stages. If you've seen a loved one inflicted with dementia, you understand how precious a year, a month, a week, or day is once the storm aims at you or a loved one.

Prolonging life in late-stage dementia without a cure amounts to cruel and unusual punishment, but patients, families, and doctors must do everything possible to extend quality of life while possible.

Make certain you have a doctor who believes in prevention and natural cures, but also remember you need their expertise concerning the best that modern medicine offers.

Be Your Nurse!

If you have a loved one, be each other's nurse. If not, be your nurse.

It's more important than ever for you to monitor your blood pressure and make notes of health issues as they arise. We don't go to the doctor every time we develop a symptom or don't feel well, but it's important to keep a medical journal. Write an outline of the problems you experience between visits.

Too often, we march into the physician's office and don't provide a full or accurate representation of our problem. For instance, if you track your blood pressure, you can furnish a pattern rather than a onetime reading. You can also perhaps attribute pikes in your blood pressure to stress taking place in your life.

You should also track other symptoms. Providing thorough information helps doctors eliminate multiple diseases with similar symptoms. When you document all or most of the symptoms that have led to the visit, you provide a competent doctor a clearer picture to develop a hypothesis. These previous unrelated symptoms might help your physician make more sense of what prompted the appointment.

Otherwise, your physician might order the wrong tests or prescribe the wrong drugs. For issues of the brain, you can't be shy or embarrassed about providing your physician with a full portrayal of your problems and symptoms.

Although still stigmatized in some circles, mental illnesses are just as real, and the sufferers are no more the blame, than physical disorders. While we must do everything in our power to avoid or slow mental or physical maladies, the last thing we need to do is embarrass those who are already suffering.

Two Dementia Series

The laborious task to document the primary dementias began as a fifty-page Alzheimer's overview. Two editions later, the 50-page Alzheimer's book turned into 400 pages.

One of the first lessons taught Alzheimer's is only one of the hundreds of diseases responsible for dementia. With inadequate testing, similar symptoms, and other handicaps, the medical community often misdiagnoses the other dementias for Alzheimer's.

My focus broadened from Alzheimer's to a dozen dementias. The only way to make any sense of Alzheimer's or dementia was to study all the primary dementias.

I worked with several neurologists and researchers over the next couple of years and hit every medical library I could hit in person or available online.

After an extensive review, I wrote the first book covering the 15 most prevalent dementia types, which provided the groundwork for two updated dementia series.

The associated *Dementia Types, Symptoms, Stages, & Risk Factors, series* expands the collection by adding amyotrophic lateral sclerosis (ALS), early-onset Alzheimer's disease, amyotrophic lateral sclerosis, corticobasal syndrome, and progressive supranuclear palsy.

Two Dementia Series

Not counting mixed dementia, there are nineteen primary dementia types, which two groundbreaking series covers.

Dementia Types, Symptoms, Stages, & Risk Factors series

1. *Dementia with Lewy Bodies*
2. *Parkinson's Disease Dementia*
3. Corticobasal Syndrome
4. Typical Alzheimer's Disease
5. *Posterior Cortical Atrophy*
6. *Down Syndrome with Alzheimer's*
7. *Limbic-predominant Age-related TDP-43 Encephalopathy (LATE)*
8. Early-onset Alzheimer's
9. *Behavioral Variant Frontotemporal Dementia*
10. Progressive Supranuclear Palsy
11. *Nonfluent Primary Progressive Aphasia*
12. Logopenic Progressive Aphasia
13. *Cortical Vascular Dementia*
14. *Binswanger Disease*
15. *Normal Pressure Hydrocephalus*
16. *Huntington's Disease*
17. *Korsakoff Syndrome*
18. *Creutzfeldt-Jakob Disease*
19. Amyotrophic Lateral Sclerosis

*Not a dementia type, but a combination, mixed dementia is the 20th category important in dementia discussions.

Any disease leading to associated symptoms is a dementia type. The series breaks medical ground by covering the dementias responsible for over 99% of dementia cases.

14

Dementia Overview Series

The second series focuses on all the primary dementia types or breaks them down as groups.

2020 Dementia Overview Series

1. Dementia Types, Symptoms, & Stages
2. *Lewy Body/Parkinsonism Dementias*
3. *Vascular Dementia*
4. *Frontotemporal Dementia (FTD)*
5. Alzheimer's Related Dementias
6. *Prevent or Slow Dementia*

The Best Science in Everyday Language

The text in both series contains American, Australian, British, and other English. I write in American English, but the research comes from the best studies worldwide. Quotes from the UK, Australia, and other English-speaking countries depend on the local dialect. For integrity, I do not edit quotes.

The books include facts and science as they exist. As much as possible, we replace medical jargon with everyday language.

Having explained the series, let's discuss dementia.

I. DEMENTIA

In this section, we discuss dementia.

Dementia is not a disease but a medical condition. Hundreds of diseases and disorders lead to dementia, but percentage-wise, almost all dementia falls under 19 primary dementia categories.

This series is the first to cover all 19 primary dementia types.

In this chapter, we answer the following questions:

- What is dementia?
- What are the 19 primary dementias?
- How prevalent is dementia?
- Who is most likely to get dementia?
- What are the financial costs to individuals, the U.S., and worldwide?

Once we answer these questions and provide a dementia overview, we turn our attention to the subject matter for the rest of the book.

Let's begin by answering the question: What is dementia?

Chapter 1: WHAT IS DEMENTIA?

For centuries, when one got dementia, people described the person in terms like "gone mad," or "lost their mind," or "crazy," or another derogatory term that missed the mark.

While most dementia types attack cognitive skills and cause behavioral disorders, the person is no less a victim than a cancer patient.

Whereas cancer attacks cells and organs, dementia destroys brain neurons.

The brain is complex. One-hundred billion neurons use over 100 trillion synapses and about 100 neurotransmitters to send all the signals to other parts of the brain, organs, and parts throughout the body, allowing us to think, reason, walk, talk, breathe, and do all that makes us human.

When fed, protected, and healthy, neurons perform magic.

The different dementias attack the brain and destroy the communication network responsible for everything our body does. By attacking different parts of the brain, the dementia types cause different disorders.

Let's see how some of the most prestigious American and global medical organizations define Dementia.

Alzheimer's Association Definition

Let's begin with the Alzheimer's Association:

> *Dementia is an overall term for diseases and conditions characterized by a decline in memory, language, problem-solving, and other thinking skills that affect a person's ability to perform everyday activities. Memory loss is an example. Alzheimer's is the most common cause of dementia[1].*

Dementia is to Alzheimer's, dementia with Lewy bodies,

Parkinson's dementia, vascular and the other dementia types what Asia is to China, India, North Korea, South Korea, and the rest of Asia. Alzheimer's is the most prevalent dementia, but each type devastates, and most are death sentences.

Let's turn to the National Institute on Aging (NIH) and see how they define dementia.

National Institute on Aging (NIH)

The National Institute on Aging (NIH) funds many studies and provides researchers invaluable data. How do they define dementia?

> *Dementia is the loss of cognitive functioning – thinking, remembering, and reasoning – and behavioral abilities to such an extent that it interferes with a person's daily life and activities. These functions include memory, language skills, visual perception, problem-solving, self-management, and the ability to focus and pay attention. Some people with dementia cannot control their emotions, and their personalities may change. Dementia ranges in severity from the mildest stage, when it is just beginning to affect a person's functioning, to the most severe stage, when the person must depend completely on others for basic activities of living*[2].

One of the most important things a person and their loved ones can do when diagnosed with dementia; enjoy what quality time remains.

Early diagnosis, medication, and lifestyle changes can slow the disease and extend quality life. From the point of diagnosis, make the most of each good day or moment.

Let's see how the international community defines dementia.

Alzheimer's Society UK

The Alzheimer's Society is perhaps the UK's most

prestigious Alzheimer's organization. They define dementia:

The word 'dementia' describes a set of symptoms that may include memory loss and difficulties with thinking, problem-solving or language. These changes are often small to start with, but for someone with dementia they have become severe enough to affect daily life. A person with dementia may also experience changes in their mood or behaviour[3].

Let's see how the World Health Organization (WHO) defines dementia.

World Health Organization (WHO)

The World Health Organization (WHO) works with global medical organizations and provides researchers a wealth of information. How does WHO define dementia?

Dementia is a syndrome – usually of a chronic or progressive nature – in which there is deterioration in cognitive function (i.e. the ability to process thought) beyond what might be expected from normal ageing. It affects memory, thinking, orientation, comprehension, calculation, learning capacity, language, and judgement. Consciousness is not affected. The impairment in cognitive function is commonly accompanied, and occasionally preceded, by deterioration in emotional control, social behaviour, or motivation[4].

The four organizations provide similar definitions, each emphasizing different points, but none contradicting the others.

Each organization confirms dementia is a broad neurological disorder. Hundreds of pathologies such as Alzheimer's leads to dementia, but 19 primary types cause about 99% of dementia cases. Dementia attacks the brain and causes memory decline, behavior disorders, motor decline, language deterioration, and most types are incurable.

If doctors diagnose you with dementia, you must get past the shock. Time is moving against you, so make the most of it.

As the Alzheimer's Society points out, the symptoms are minor in the beginning. Get your affairs in order, enjoy loved ones, and take part in as many activities as you desire and are able. To some extent, this is your farewell tour. Take advantage!

The disease will stop you or a loved one later, so do not stop living your life in the early stages.

Let's next examine the 19 primary dementia types.

Chapter 2: WHAT ARE THE 19 PRIMARY DEMENTIAS?

Hundreds of medical conditions lead to dementia, but 19 causes up to 99% of cases.

Each dementia type is devastating, most are fatal, and the first symptoms to death is a challenging, heartbreaking, soul-crushing experience. Dementia robs the personalities and functionality of marvelous people a little at a time until they no longer resemble the person they've always been.

19 Dementia Types

This chapter divides the 19 primary dementias into six categories. The first group includes dementias related to Lewy body or Parkinsonism dementia. The second consists of Alzheimer's-related dementia. In the third, we focus on primary progressive aphasia dementias. The fourth contains vascular dementias. The fifth category encompasses the remaining dementias and is called *other dementias*.

Lewy Body/Parkinsonism Related Dementias

1. *Dementia with Lewy Bodies*
2. *Parkinson's Disease Dementia*
3. Corticobasal Syndrome

Alzheimer's Related Dementias

4. Typical Alzheimer's Disease
5. *Posterior Cortical Atrophy*
6. *Down Syndrome with Alzheimer's*
7. *Limbic-predominant Age-related TDP-43 Encephalopathy (LATE)*
8. Early-onset Alzheimer's

Frontotemporal Lobar Degeneration Related Dementias

9. *Behavioral Variant Frontotemporal Dementia*
10. Progressive Supranuclear Palsy

Primary Progressive Aphasia Related Dementias

11. *Nonfluent Primary Progressive Aphasia (nfvPPA)*
12. Logopenic Progressive Aphasia (LPA)

Vascular Dementia

13. *Cortical Vascular Dementia*
14. *Binswanger Disease*

Other Dementias

15. *Normal Pressure Hydrocephalus*
16. *Huntington's Disease*
17. *Korsakoff Syndrome*
18. *Creutzfeldt-Jakob Disease*
19. Amyotrophic Lateral Sclerosis

Chapter 3: WHO IS MOST LIKELY TO GET DEMENTIA?

In this chapter, we explore who is most likely to get dementia. Most know people with dementia are old, but some people are born with dementia, others get it as infants, and the disease attacks people in every age group.

There are risk factors that affect everybody. Examples include a poor diet, lack of exercise, diabetes, obesity, high blood pressure, and factors under and beyond our control.

In this chapter, we focus on risk factors affecting specific groups of people who suffer higher rates.

The research pointed to age, race, and sex, where dementia seems to discriminate. Let's review the science for each.

Age

Age is the obvious risk factor. We know because of science and our observations.

So associated with the elderly, many believe dementia only strikes older people. However, dementia strikes all ages and demographics, including newborns and infants.

According to Stanford University Medical School, "The risk of Alzheimer's disease, vascular dementia, and several other dementias goes up significantly with advancing age[5]."

None of us enjoy aging. We must work harder and harder to slow aging, and no matter how well we do, none of us will make it much past 100 years. The better we take care of ourselves, the higher chance we have of living a quality life into our eighties or nineties.

Remember, aging does not destroy our cognitive abilities. Bad habits do! I stress this point because each of us can slow the aging process through healthy habits.

As people age, however, our dementia risks increase.

A Journal of Neurology, Neurosurgery, & Psychiatry study

concluded[6]:

> *In the age group 65–69 years, there are more than two new cases per 1000 persons every year. This number increases almost exponentially with increasing age, until over the age of 90 years, out of 1000 persons, 70 new cases of dementia can be expected every year.*

As we stress in our book on prevention, there is actual age and real age. We determine one's actual age by the day and year born, whereas weight, blood pressure, blood sugar, cholesterol, diet, how often you work out, and several other important factors govern our real age.

Unless genes or an accident prevents us, our real age should be lower than our actual age. Those who practice bad habits, however, raise their real age ten years or more than their actual age.

When our real age is lower than our actual age, we lower our risks for dementia and other diseases. When our real age is higher than our actual age, we increase risks for dementia, heart disease, cancer, and all major diseases.

Let's next review if race plays a role in dementia.

Race

African Americans and blacks in western countries suffer more than their share of racism.

The United States has abused too many citizens since its creation, but none more than Native Americans and African Americans.

But, does dementia also discriminate against them?

According to AARP, African Americans are 64% more likely to get dementia than non-Hispanic whites[7].

Kaiser Permanente Study

Researchers in another study examined data from 274,000

Kaiser Permanente patients over 14 years. They found the highest rate of dementia for African Americans and Native Americans[8].

Dementia Risk Per 1,000 People

- 27 African Americans
- 22 Native Americans
- 20 Latinos and Pacific Islanders
- 19 White Americans
- 15 Asian-Americans

Does dementia love Asian and European-Americans and hate African and Native-Americans?

Dementia is as evil as the worst bigot, but dementia is not a bigot.

African Americans experience higher rates of diabetes. African Americans and Native Americans suffer a higher level of stress, poverty, and disenfranchisement. Both cultures also struggle with their people's history in European-America and endure a greater level of bigotry and more obstacles to succeeding in modern America.

On the flip side, Asian Americans and whites have lower obesity and diabetes rates, eat a more balanced diet, faceless bigotry, are more affluent, educated, and successful in modern America.

We need more studies to confirm the exact causes of higher dementia incidence in the African and Native American populations. Higher stress and diabetes in their communities are prime suspects.

Jennifer Manly, Columbia University, Taub Institute for Research on Alzheimer's disease, and Aging Brain spoke to Reuters about the inequities.

> *There are huge disparities in dementia that*
> *are confronting this nation and this will*
> *translate into an enormous burden on families if*

we don't address this. We need to prioritize research that uncovers the reasons for these disparities and more research should include racially and ethnically diverse people[9].

Are African British at a greater risk for Dementia?

In the United Kingdom, black women are 25% more likely than white women, and black men 28% more likely than white men to get dementia[10].

Reluctance to Take Part in Dementia Studies

African Americans and Native Americans are also less trustful of studies. Too often in the past, a bigoted establishment treated African Americans and Native Americans like lab rats.

The awful past makes the average African American reluctant to take part in studies that might help us figure out how to lower the rates.

Native Americans are also distrustful of the United States government and the "white man's studies," as one group from the Cherokee Reservation in North Carolina told me.

I understand both ethnic groups' skepticism. As somebody with ancestors who died and survived the Trail of Tears, and who married a black woman (30+ years), nobody must convince me of the tainted American history. I have read about the past and viewed enough with my own eyes to know the sins of America's past, either haunt or still torment today.

But, the Studies are Necessary!

I call on African Americans and Native Americans to take part in dementia studies. The studies today have greater safeguards than the past and face much more scrutiny.

Dementia is a death sentence!

Worse than the average killer, never content to kill and move on, dementia is a sadist. Dementia destroys the mind and body, little by little, robbing one's personality, dignity, mind, body, and everything that makes a person unique.

If African Americans and Native Americans refuse to participate in dementia studies, fatal neurological disorders will continue to strike them worse than other ethnic groups.

Please consider two facts.

If you do not have dementia, researchers do not subject you to drug trials but accumulate data to determine which habits increase and decrease one's risks.

If doctors diagnose you with dementia, trials represent your last best chance to win what is otherwise a losing battle.

What Role does Poverty Play?

Although not listed as a dementia risk factor, poverty increases one's risk for almost every significant disease. Those at the bottom must worry where the next meal is coming, if somebody might mug (or kill) them when leaving the house, and a laundry list of stress the average citizen seems oblivious.

Beller Health calls for more research to determine if Native American, African American, and African British citizens have higher dementia rates as a general population, or if poverty drives these numbers. We need to know whether the number also applies to middle-and upper-class African Americans and Native Americans who eat healthily, exercise, do not abuse alcohol, avoid tobacco, and do not abuse prescription or illicit drugs.

Native American, African American, and African British citizens suffer a higher percentage of poverty than other demographics in the US and UK.

Rather than race, such factors as poverty, bigotry, and lack of opportunities might drive these numbers.

I reached out to several organizations, including the VA, to conduct a large-scale study to determine what role poverty plays in dementia. Most organizations greeted my request with enthusiasm, and I hope one or more soon back the study.

All we know for certain is poverty in the industrial world causes a much greater level of stress and other hardships than the rest of the population. WHO reported that about 60% of dementia cases occur in the poorest half of countries[11].

Age and ethnicity are dementia risk factors. What about sex?

Sex

Dementia strikes older people, African Americans, Native Americans, and African British in greater numbers than the rest of the population. Does one's gender increase or decrease one's odds?

How Many Women have Dementia?

According to the Alzheimer's Association, women represent two-thirds of people living with Alzheimer's, and 13 million women suffer dementia or are caring for somebody who does[12].

Of the 820,000 people living with dementia in the UK, females account for 61 percent[13].

Of the 50 million people living with dementia worldwide[14], women represent 65 percent[15].

Key points:

- Women represent two-thirds of Alzheimer's cases.
- Females account for 65% of dementia cases.

Is dementia just another woman-hating predator?

Does Alzheimer's & Most Dementia Strike Women in Greater Numbers?

While the two key numbers suggest dementia is a rampaging woman-abusing murderer, the answer is not so simple.

While women represent two-thirds of Alzheimer's cases and 65% of dementia cases, there are 19 primary dementia types.

Some dementias attack men in greater numbers and much harder than females. The dementias we know attack men in greater ratios include[16]:

- Parkinson's dementia (Lewy body dementia)
- Dementia with Lewy bodies (Lewy body dementia)
- Post-Stroke dementia (Vascular dementia)

28

- Multi-infarct dementia (Vascular dementia)
- Binswanger Disease(Vascular dementia)
- Normal pressure hydrocephalus
- Behavioral variant frontotemporal dementia
- Primary Progressive Aphasia (Frontotemporal dementia)
- Chronic traumatic encephalopathy
- HIV-related cognitive impairment
- Amyotrophic lateral sclerosis

From the data about the 19 primary dementias, at least eleven attack men in greater numbers. Data is not available for Creutzfeldt-Jakob disease, Wernicke-Korsakoff Syndrome, LATE, and Down syndrome with Alzheimer's disease. The remaining dementias strike both genders in similar numbers. When the authorities release more information, we will update this section.

If a minimum of 11 of 19 dementia types strike men in greater numbers than women, how can 68% of people living with dementia be women?

Alzheimer's accounts for 60-80% of dementia, and two-thirds of people with Alzheimer's are women.

When we say dementia attacks, women, 65% to 35% men, we distort the picture. I call on the medical community to provide greater clarity. More precise, we should warn women to represent two-thirds of total Alzheimer's cases, but stress a minimum of 11 of 19 dementia types strike men in greater numbers.

Treating dementia and Alzheimer's as interchangeable terms is misleading. There are 19 primary dementias and 11 or more attack men in greater numbers. If we exclude Alzheimer's and focus on the other 18 primary dementia types, they attack men by far greater percentages.

With that stipulation, let's explore why Alzheimer's and some dementias attack women more than men.

Why Does Alzheimer's & Dementia Strike Women in Greater Numbers Than Men?

In part, unique burdens & responsibilities explain the disparity.

Women still fight today for equality. Like Native Americans, African Americans, and African British, the average woman carries burdens; the average man is clueless.

To be a woman, one fights for equality from birth in a "man's world," as the song and tradition attest. Among things unique to women:

- Menstrual cycles (ranging from mild to horrendous)
- Childbirth
- Menopause

Being a guy is also difficult, but there's no denying women are born with unique responsibilities and burdens.

As an aunt once retorted, if they live long enough, every woman suffers menstrual cycles until menopause "tortures it out."

Women Live Longer

Women outlive men in the United States and worldwide.

Worldwide, the average man lives to age 69.8, while the average woman lives 74.2 years[17]. These are the average numbers, so they fluctuate from region to region and country to country.

Let's see how these numbers compare to the United States.

American Comparisons

The CDC reports the average American male lives 76 years, compared to the average American woman who lives 81 years[18].

Why Do Women Live Longer Than Men?

Although women live longer, this might result because

more men abuse alcohol, tobacco, and drugs, get less sleep, work in more hazardous jobs, suffer greater casualties in war, and take unnecessary risks.

The lead author of a study published in the *British Medical Journal*, Australian neuropsychiatrist Richard Cibulskis, confirmed some of my suspicions.

> *Men are much more likely to die from preventable and treatable non-communicable diseases, such as {ischemic} heart disease and lung cancer, and road traffic accidents*[19].

Global population expert, Dr. Perminder Sachdev, confirmed my other suspicions in an interview with *Time*.

"Men are more likely to smoke, drink excessively and be overweight," Sachdev said. "They are also less likely to seek medical help early, and, if diagnosed with a disease, they are more likely to be non-adherent to treatment." Sachdev also pointed out, "men are more likely to take life-threatening risks and to die in car accidents, brawls or gunfights[20]."

Although nature perhaps installed a natural order to preserve the female population, men's reckless nature might account for the five years difference in life expectancy between the genders.

It will interest to see if the numbers change as more women become more like men. Women are assuming greater roles in war, law enforcement, and other areas where even men with healthy habits have fallen. As the societal lines between men and women blur, the difference in life expectancy should fall.

In all honorable fields of life, women should go for it. Never has there been a better time to prove the equality of the sexes.

As far as men's bad habits, my hope is women continue to show better judgment and exercise greater restraint. Women will never prove their equality by emulating men's worse habits or trying to outdo us in the stupid department.

The best men and women rise on similar foundations. However, the worst men and women also share a foundation.

My hope for humans getting our act together soon hinges on the average woman being better than the average man.

Love yourselves for your unique feminine qualities. Be equal, but please do not confuse out-drinking, out-smoking, out-drugging, acting more reckless, and stupid than men with being equal. We need fewer men like that, not more women!

Chapter 4: DEMENTIA COSTS & PREVALENCE

In this chapter, we review dementia prevalence and costs to governments, the world, caregivers, and patients.

How Many People Worldwide Suffer Dementia?

According to the World Health Organization (WHO), over 50 million people suffer dementia worldwide, with 10 million new cases each year[21].

How Many Americans Have Dementia?

In the United States, 5.8 million Americans live with dementia[22], with Alzheimer's representing 70% of cases.

Let's check the UK dementia numbers.

How Many People In The UK Have Dementia?

According to the Alzheimer's Society, 850,000 people in the UK live with dementia[23].

Alzheimer's Society reports that about 70% of those living in UK care homes suffer dementia.

The numbers show Americans, British, and global citizens suffering high rates of dementia. Let's see which countries' dementia strikes the hardest.

Which Countries Have The Highest Dementia Rate?

Per World Atlas, the following ten countries suffer the highest dementia rate of deaths per 100,000 people[24]:

1. Finland
2. USA
3. Canada
4. Iceland
5. Sweden
6. Switzerland
7. Norway
8. Denmark
9. The Netherlands
10. Belgium

As we review the list, per population, dementia strikes Americans in greater numbers than any country but Finland.

Why?

There are several explanations:

- Over two-thirds of Americans are obese or overweight.
- The other countries on the list also suffer higher obesity levels than most countries not on the list.
- Because of weight issues, the countries in question suffer high rates of diabetes and high blood pressure, both dementia risk factors.
- Americans consume more prescription drugs than people worldwide. While there is no data to confirm, I suspect the other countries on the list also have greater access and use more prescription drugs than poorer countries.
- They load the western diet with salt, sugar, and

white processed flours.

- The average person in western countries lives longer than those in poorer nations.
- We will add other factors once data becomes available.
- People live longer in these countries than most not on the list (the older one lives, the greater the dementia risk)

Another explanation is more misdiagnosis and no-diagnosis in poorer countries around the world. Obesity and other risk factors are also less of a problem in developing countries.

I recommend global researchers compare the ten countries on this list. By viewing the similarities between the ten, we might better pinpoint the cause for Alzheimer's and the other dementias.

If we can figure out what the citizens from the ten nations are doing wrong, we can find the cause and means of preventing dementia. While I pointed to some of the most obvious risk factors, the most important common risk factor from the ten nations might be something unexpected.

Let's now examine dementia costs.

Dementia Costs

In this chapter, we analyze dementia costs. We examine the United States and global costs, then provide estimated costs per family.

What Does Dementia Cost the United States?

More than the entire economies of Finland and 166 other countries, dementia costs the United States $277 billion per year.

What Does Dementia Cost Worldwide?

Getting credible global numbers proves difficult, if not impossible, in any medical research. Often, the best source is the World Health Organization (WHO). They collect data from around the world and are an essential source for medical researchers.

Getting accurate dementia numbers in richer countries is difficult. In the United States and the UK, black people hesitate to take part in dementia studies or to seek medical attention for symptoms.

In richer countries, there are still too many misdiagnoses.

Thus, if we cannot get ironclad numbers in the United States, the United Kingdom, and the industrial nations, the task proves even more difficult for developing countries.

If the United States and the United Kingdom have difficulty convincing black citizens to seek medical attention for dementia symptoms, the third world faces even greater obstacles.

In the third world, most areas do well to offer their citizens basic medical care. With no urine or blood test, many regions lack resources for CAT scans, MRIs, and other expensive imaging equipment to make a diagnosis.

Without urine or blood tests, diagnosing dementia costs more than low-income people with inadequate or no insurance can afford in the richest countries.

In the United States and industrial nations, doctors often misdiagnose the other 19 primary dementias for Alzheimer's or each other.

Expecting doctors in many third world nations to diagnose dementia with inferior or no equipment is to expect miracles. If it overwhelms medical professionals in the wealthier nations, we often expect third world doctors to perform miracles. What amazes is they often do!

However, no matter how good a job the average third world doctor does treating typical medical conditions, even if trained, it does not equip them to diagnose dementia early, if at all. My comments are not criticism.

The average doctor's job is not to diagnose or treat dementia, but they must recognize symptoms and refer the patient to neurologists. Primary care physicians are the first line of defense.

North, south, east, west, dementia overwhelms the medical community.

Having discussed the limitations, let's examine the data. While the numbers are ballpark figures, landing in the park is the keystone to estimation. In most cases, the real numbers are much higher.

According to the *World Alzheimer's Report,* global dementia costs a minimum of $1 trillion per year, and experts predict it will reach $2 trillion by 2030 if we find no cure[25].

Authorities should release new numbers over the next year, and we will update this section.

The *Alzheimer's Report* global cost estimations do not include informal care costs; another reason we consider the estimates conservative.

The Alzheimer's Report concluded:

> *Direct medical care costs account for roughly 20% of global dementia costs, while direct social sector costs and informal care costs each account for roughly 40%. The relative contribution of informal care is greatest in the African regions and lowest in North America, Western Europe and some South American regions, while the reverse is true for social sector costs.*

Whatever the real up-to-date costs, we must take action to reduce the burden on individuals and nations. If we do not invest in independent research to develop an effective urine or blood test, cure, and vaccine for each dementia type, the costs will smother economies throughout the world. The costs will cripple developing countries and destabilize the wealthiest.

We have no choice but to invest more in dementia research. No matter which country you live, your economy, security, and the health of your nation rides on us finding a cure or vaccine.

As a scientist, I find it disturbing climate change and independent dementia research are not major priorities. Most governments, businesses, and individuals who can afford to fund dementia remain MIA in the war against dementia.

Before we conclude this section, let's examine the dementia statistics side-by-side in the table below.

DEMENTIA STATISTICS

This table focuses on the number of people with dementia and the number of deaths per 100,000 among the nations chosen for comparison.

NATION	# OF PEOPLE WITH DEMENTIA	DEMENTIA DEATHS PER 100,000 PEOPLE	TOTAL COSTS (US DOLLARS)
Australia	447,115	29.61	$15 billion
Brazil	1 million +	10.71	$16.45 billion
Canadian	747,000	37.30	$10.4 billion
China	16.93 million	19.87	$69 billion
France	1.2 million	30.84	$37.91 billion
Germany	1.5 million	16.99	$57.57 billion
India	4 million	14.57	$28.38 billion
Italy	1.4 million	19.81	$29.96 billion
Japan	4.6 million	7.22	$14.8 billion
Mexico	800,000	3.62	Not available
Spain	800.000+	29.23	$19.98 million
Netherlands	280,000	39.37	$4.44 million
United States	5.8 million	44.41	$290 billion
United Kingdom	850,000	49.18	$26.3 billion

Sources: World Health Rankings[26], Alzheimer's Europe[27], NATSIM[28], Alzheimer's Society[29], Brain Test[30]

Other sources cited in the chapter.

The table comes from my book <u>2020 Dementia Overview</u>, which covers cost and prevalence among comparative nations in greater detail.

Let's next discuss the dementia costs for caregivers.

What Does Dementia Cost Volunteer Caregivers?

Although 41% make less than $50,000, American voluntary caregivers devote a minimum of 18.4 billion hours per year to dementia patients.

Worth $232 billion per year, we underrate the voluntary caregiving heroes in our fight against dementia. This total does not include lost wages for the voluntary caregiver.

According to the Northwestern Mutual C.A.R.E. Study, 67% of voluntary caregivers must cut their living to help pay for the patient's medical care, and 57% end up experiencing financial problems[31].

Adding to the costs of voluntary caregivers, they often end up sick themselves. Caring for loved ones with dementia bankrupts many.

In the early stages, the loved one can still perform most of their daily tasks but will require 24/7 care once the symptoms advance.

Imagine putting your life on hold for years to care, bathe, feed, protect, and take such a heavy load on your shoulders.

Millions of dementia families face the dilemma where the husband and wife both must work in most families to get by. You work as a couple to build stability in your own family, and then, boom, doctors diagnose one of you with dementia.

What Does Dementia Cost Dementia Patients?

When we say patient, past a certain stage in the disease, we refer to family or loved ones. A person who cannot perform daily tasks cannot manage finances, even if they have any left.

Too often, the costs drive entire families into bankruptcy because of dementia costs for a member.

Authorities estimate the average cost per dementia patient is $341,840, with families expected to cover 70 percent.

The costs devastate the average family in the industrial nations.

How are they supposed to afford it in developing countries where the average citizen makes less than one-thousand American dollars per year?

Dementia Recap

Although your dementia research has just begun, you now have a decent overview of Dementia.

In Chapter One, we explored dementia. We turned to several top dementia or medical organizations and compared their definitions.

Chapter two explained Alzheimer's is to dementia what China is to Asia. We listed the 19 dementias.

19 Primary Dementia Types

Why is it important to learn about the most prevalent dementias?

There are several reasons. One, the dementias share similar symptoms and—with no accurate testing—doctors often misdiagnose for one of a hundred or more other possibilities. Two, if a person gets one dementia, more often than not, they develop an overlapping second dementia type, known as mixed dementia. In some cases, three dementia types might develop in later stages.

The pathology, related-proteins, atrophy location, and the resulting symptoms determine dementia classifications.

The more we learn about dementia, dementia types, and subtypes grow.

We once thought of Alzheimer's disease as one sweeping neurological disorder, but now know there is typical Alzheimer's, behavior variant Alzheimer's, posterior cortical atrophy, Early-onset Alzheimer's, and the newest dementia category, LATE, previously misdiagnosed for typical Alzheimer's. If that is not complicated enough, there are 20-40 typical Alzheimer's types.

Depending on the pathology, the three primary progressive aphasia subtypes are either Alzheimer's or frontotemporal-related.

We know there is not one vascular dementia, but three: post-stroke dementia, multi-infarct dementia, and Binswanger disease.

There are two Lewy body dementias; Parkinson's disease dementia and dementia with Lewy bodies. There are also other Parkinson-related neurological disorders.

Lewy Body/Parkinsonism Related Dementias

1. *Dementia with Lewy Bodies*
2. *Parkinson's Disease Dementia*
3. Corticobasal Syndrome

Alzheimer's Related Dementias

4. Typical Alzheimer's Disease
5. *Posterior Cortical Atrophy*
6. *Down Syndrome with Alzheimer's*
20. *Limbic-predominant Age-related TDP-43 Encephalopathy (LATE)*
7. Early-onset Alzheimer's

Frontotemporal Lobar Degeneration Related Dementias

8. *Behavioral Variant Frontotemporal Dementia*
9. Progressive Supranuclear Palsy

Primary Progressive Aphasia Related Dementias

10. *Nonfluent Primary Progressive Aphasia (nfvPPA)*
11. Logopenic Progressive Aphasia (LPA)

Vascular Dementia

12. *Cortical Vascular Dementia*
13. *Binswanger Disease*

Other Dementias

14. *Normal Pressure Hydrocephalus*
15. *Huntington's Disease*
16. *Korsakoff Syndrome*
17. *Creutzfeldt-Jakob Disease*
18. Amyotrophic Lateral Sclerosis

Although most the dementia types share similar symptoms, enough to cause misdiagnosis, each has its unique pathology and symptoms.

In chapter three, we explored dementia prevalence in the United States, the UK, and worldwide.

Chapter four examined who is most likely to get dementia. We found Native Americans (those who greeted the first Europeans), and black citizens in the United States and the UK are more likely to get dementia than their white or Asian counterparts.

We also explored the women to men ratio. Women represent two-thirds of Alzheimer's and over sixty percent of dementia cases. We pointed out the Alzheimer's figure skews the dementia numbers because men are more likely to get a minimum of 11 of the 19 primary dementia types.

Chapter four explored the US, UK, global, patient, family, and voluntary caregivers' dementia costs. The staggering numbers are almost as frightening as the medical disorder itself.

Dementia Costs & Prevalence

NATION	# OF PEOPLE WITH DEMENTIA	DEMENTIA DEATHS PER 100,000 PEOPLE	TOTAL COSTS (US DOLLARS)
Australia	447,115	29.61	$15 billion
Brazil	1 million +	10.71	$16.45 billion
Canadian	747,000	37.30	$10.4 billion
China	16.93 million	19.87	$69 billion
France	1.2 million	30.84	$37.91 billion
Germany	1.5 million	16.99	$57.57 billion
India	4 million	14.57	$28.38 billion
Italy	1.4 million	19.81	$29.96 billion
Japan	4.6 million	7.22	$14.8 billion
Mexico	800,000	3.62	Not available
Spain	800.000+	29.23	$19.98 million
Netherlands	280,000	39.37	$4.44 million
United States	5.8 million	44.41	$290 billion
United Kingdom	850,000	49.18	$26.3 billion

Sources: World Health Rankings[32], Alzheimer's Europe[33], NATSIM[34], Alzheimer's Society[35], Brain Test[36]

The table comes from 2020 Dementia Overview, which covers cost and prevalence among comparative nations in greater detail.

After reviewing the conservative numbers, and factoring in an aging population, we concluded we must find a cure before it bankrupts millions of families and cripples nations.

Let's turn our attention to this book's subject, Lewy body, and Parkinsonism dementias.

II. LEWY BODY (LBD)/PARKINSONS-RELATED DEMENTIAS

1. Dementia with Lewy Bodies
2. Parkinson's Disease Dementia
3. Corticobasal Syndrome

Chapter 5: WHAT IS LEWY BODY DEMENTIA (LBD)?

People in their late teens and early twenties make some of the greatest discoveries. When 26, Albert Einstein released (then) groundbreaking scientific papers on Brownian motion, special relativity, photoelectric effect, and the equivalence of mass and energy.

When his doctor-father complained about the limitations of the echocardiogram, 15-year-old Suman Mulumudi used a 3-D printer to develop the Steth IO, which provides better sound than the stethoscope and comes with a visual graph. At 22, Galileo published a book outlining his design of hydrostatic balance. At age 16, in 1642, Blaise Pascal developed the first calculating devices and prototypes leading to the computer revolution.

A young person also discovered Lewy body dementia.

In 1912, German Dr. Friedrich H. Lewy[37] discovered Lewy body dementia (LBD) while analyzing Parkinson's disease[38].

Although later persecuted as a Jew (he and wife fled to the United States during W.W. II), Dr. Lewy discovered Lewy body dementia only two years after completing medical school. Dr. Lewy is a testament to not only what young people can accomplish, but also how a person can overcome great hardship.

Please view the image below to see how Lewy bodies form in the brain.

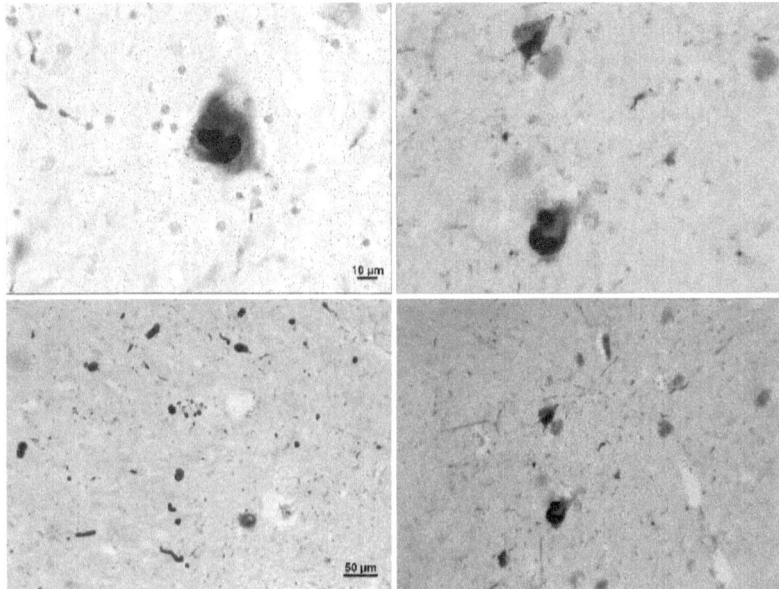

Lewy Body[39]

The spots in the image represent the Lewy bodies or alpha synuclein protein forming on the brain. As we soon discuss, alpha synuclein plays a vital role in our mental health, but something unknown makes the brain produce too much.

The deposits cause dementia with Lewy bodies and are responsible for Parkinson's disease patients who also suffer dementia in later stages.

Let's investigate what is Lewy body dementia (LBD), if there is a cure, and what causes LBD.

What is Lewy Body Dementia (LBD)?

Protein buildups are prevalent in most dementias, and Lewy body dementia (LBD) is no different.

"Protein deposits, called Lewy bodies," said the Mayo Clinic, "develop in nerve cells in the brain regions involved in thinking, memory and movement[40] (motor control)."

The Lewy Body Association[41] provides a similar definition.

Lewy body dementia (LBD) is a progressive brain disorder in which Lewy bodies (abnormal deposits of a protein called alpha-synuclein) build up in areas of the brain that regulate behavior, cognition, and movement.

Be it amyloid, tau, or some other form, a protein's relationship to Alzheimer's, Vascular dementia, and other dementias are the root of the problem. In Lewy body dementia, we focus on alpha synuclein protein.

Is there a cure for Lewy body dementia?

Like most dementias, there is no cure to Lewy body dementia, but early detection remains important to slow and treat symptoms[42]. To find a cure, we need governments and corporations to invest more in independent research to discover tests, vaccines, and cures for each of the primary dementias.

While no cure exists, there is much we can do to prevent this and other dementias.

What causes Lewy body dementia?

Science does not know what causes LBD but focuses on a protein buildup, alpha synuclein, that clumps into Lewy bodies.

Alpha-Synuclein

Another trademark of protein related to dementias, researchers from the University of California San Francisco Medical Center, confirmed alpha synuclein is a double-edged sword.

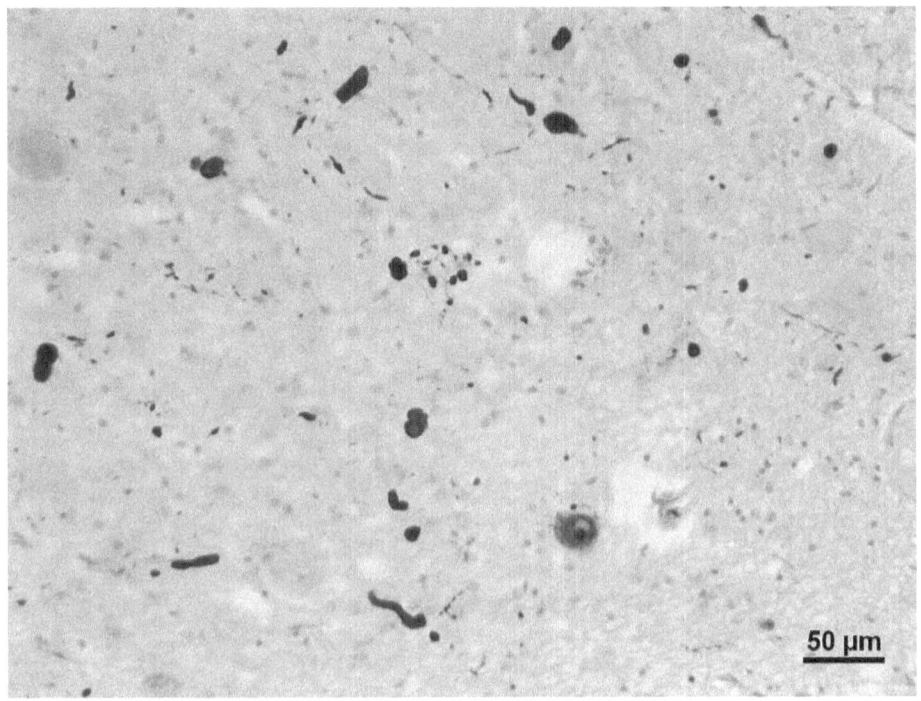

Lewy bodies (alpha synuclein inclusions) [43]

The study's lead author Robert Edwards, M.D., discussed the results. High levels of Lewy bodies (alpha synuclein) present in Parkinson's disease inhibits fusion between vesicles and membranes, "necessary for neurotransmitter release," said Edwards. "But in normal amounts, it has a surprisingly different effect: if neurotransmitters are already being released, alpha-synuclein helps speed the process[44]."

Scientists must learn if the protein forms to protect the neurons, or mutated genes destroy the neuron network related to many motor and non-motor skills.

Several neurologists, including Dale Bredesen and David Perlmutter, argue the overactive proteins are an effect not cause. According to them, the protein deposits associated with dementias such as Alzheimer's are protective mechanisms in response to true causes such as viruses like herpes, oral infections, toxins, and inflammation.

If true, this explains why all dementia drug trials failed up to this point. By focusing on the true causes, researchers stand a better chance of developing tests, vaccines, and cures for each dementia type, including Lewy body dementias.

Lewy Bodies

Lewy bodies result when alpha synuclein protein develops clumps and deposits. Alpha synuclein forms in the brain stem and clumps cause "resting tremor," slowness, and stiffness.

The protein clumps kill neurons and the brain's elaborate communication system, causing Lewy body dementia symptoms.

The deposits can also affect the cortex area of the brain and inhibit cognitive skills. We soon discuss the symptoms the deposits produce.

Please examine the brain's cortex in the image below.

Cortex

The cortex is the outside layer of the brain inhabited by millions of neurons[45]. When many think of the brain, they form an image of the cortex.

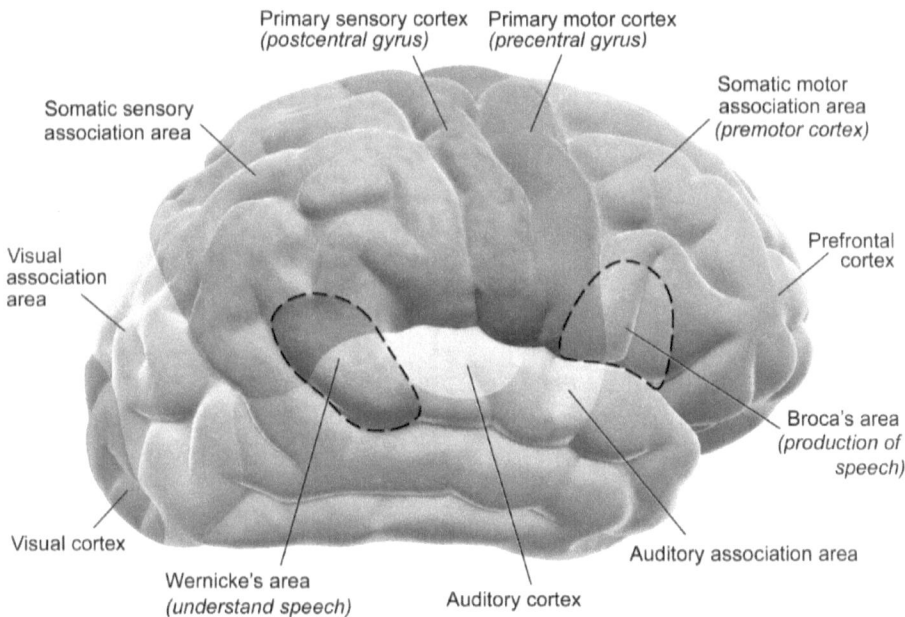

Source[46]: "Medical gallery of Blausen Medical 2014,"

The brain depends on the cortex for sensory skills. Let's discuss the seven cortex areas.

7 Cortex Areas

1. Primary visual cortex is in the occipital lobe[47]
2. Primary auditory cortex above the temporal lobe[48]
3. Primary somatosensory cortex is behind the central sulcus[49]
4. Secondary somatosensory cortex by the lateral fissure[50]
5. Primary motor cortex sits in front of the primary somatosensory cortex[51]
6. Premotor cortex resides in the section on the motor cortex in the frontal lobe[52]
7. Pre-frontal cortex locates in front of pre-motor cortex[53]

The different layers of cortex and the neurons within manage our movement and cognitive skills. When the protein deposits damage the neurons, our sensory and motor skills breakdown.

We revisit these topics in the chapters on symptoms and stages.

Lewy Body dementia is a medical condition reached from opposite directions, named Parkinson's disease dementia (PDD) and dementia with Lewy bodies (DLB).

Two Lewy Body Dementia (LBD) Types

There are two versions of Lewy body dementia:

1. Dementia with Lewy bodies (DLB)
2. Parkinson's disease dementia (PDD)

Dementia with Lewy bodies and PDD pose opposite routes to the same neurological disorder.

The University of California, San Francisco, provides an informative overview:

> *Lewy body dementias include dementia with Lewy bodies (DLB) and Parkinson's disease with dementia (PDD) and are the second most frequent cause of dementia in elderly adults. These degenerative brain diseases are associated with abnormal clumps of a protein called alpha-synuclein. These clumps, called Lewy bodies, are found in nerve cells throughout the outer layer of the brain (the cerebral cortex) and deep inside the midbrain and brainstem. Patients with these diseases experience progressive cognitive decline, although there is considerable variability in symptoms between patients. Common symptoms include problems with movement, visual hallucinations, and fluctuations in thinking skills or attention[54].*

According to John Hopkins Health Library[55], over 1.4 million Americans suffer one of the two forms of Lewy body dementia[56].

Misdiagnosis

Lewy Body Dementia Association (LBDA) warns that many doctors are unaware or don't understand Lewy body dementia, and misdiagnose many patients who go untreated, under-treated, or maltreated.

Compared to past generations, there's much more information today, a primary care physician must learn. I also stress it is no fault to primary care physicians; there is no accurate blood or urine test for dementia as there is for cancer and other diseases (Hello Congress!).

Note to Doctors & Medical Professionals

When treating Parkinson's-like symptoms, doctors should resist the urge to prescribe antipsychotic drugs. According to LBDA, such drugs cause neuroleptic malignant syndrome in people who have dementia with Lewy bodies or Parkinson's related dementia[57].

The combination of misdiagnosis and the resulting antipsychotic medication shut down kidneys and speeds up the most devastating effects of dementia, including death. That is if one doesn't die when the kidneys shut down.

Note to Patients

Choosing the right doctor is more important than ever. Being medical-book-smart is not enough to diagnose and treat dementia because the medical books remain incomplete on the subject.

To diagnose dementia, one must never stop learning and do their best to keep up and make sense of the endless important medical studies on all diseases doctors treat.

The dementia deck is stacked against the primary care physician and challenges the best neurologists. You must be the first care provider for your health.

Help the doctor and medical officials by documenting your symptoms, making a doctor's appointment as soon as neurological symptoms develop, and help them fill in the pieces to the puzzle.

Patients trust doctors to make most dementia-related decisions with an incomplete handbook. Besides diagnosing and treating hundreds of other potential medical issues their patients face, doctors must tread through mountains and valleys of conflicting dementia information.

Without accurate urine or blood tests for most dementias, we're expecting the impossible from primary care physicians.

That doctors already are fighting dementia without enough tools makes it even more important you find a doctor you trust with your life.

Misdiagnosis is not simply a matter of having or not having money, having or not having good insurance—although those are factors. Diagnosing dementia is a guessing game, guaranteeing widespread misdiagnosis.

When Robin Williams died, news outlets reported depression drove him to suicide. However, his autopsy showed Williams suffered Lewy body dementia, which had gone undiagnosed.

Doctors diagnosed and treated Robin Williams for Parkinson's disease, but only the autopsy confirmed the Lewy bodies had spread through his brain, evidence to Lewy body dementia.

Even after the autopsy, specialists debate whether Williams had dementia with Lewy bodies or Parkinson's disease dementia.

Dennis Dickson, M.D., Mayo Clinic, and a member of the LBDA Scientific Advisory Council analyzed the coroner's report.

"Mr. Williams was given a clinical diagnosis of PD and treated for motor symptoms," said Dr. Dickson. "The report confirms he experienced depression, anxiety, and paranoia, which may occur in either Parkinson's disease or dementia with Lewy bodies."

If a wealthy and famous actor such as Robin Williams falls through the cracks, the rest of us can too. I am not accusing Robin Williams' doctors of negligence, but complain again we do not have a simple, accurate test or cure for Parkinson's disease, Parkinson's disease dementia, dementia with Lewy bodies, Alzheimer's disease and most dementias.

The governments of the world should be ashamed for not supporting and funding the research for scientists to conduct the studies to develop an accurate and cheap test and cure for these devastating diseases.

What Is The Difference Between Dementia With Lewy Bodies (DLB) And Parkinson's Disease Dementia (PDD)?

Dementia with Lewy bodies (DLB) and Parkinson's disease dementia (PDD) are two paths to Lewy body Dementia (LBD).

A *Fifth Department of Internal Medicine* study explains it is difficult to distinguish between DLB and PDD, except dementia strikes before Parkinsonism in the former, whereas Parkinsonism predates dementia in the latter. Otherwise, "there are few or no pathological differences between DLB and PDD," according to the Fukuoka University study[58].

Ester Heerema, MSW, and Claudia Chaves, MD, explain why it is difficult to distinguish between dementia with Lewy bodies and Parkinson's disease with dementia. "Symptoms that affect the body include muscle weakness, rigidity (stiffness), and slowness in movements," said Heerema. "Symptoms in the brain include impaired executive functioning, attention span, and memory loss."

Patients with DLB and PDD both suffer from depression and hallucinations.

Are they different versions of the same disease, as some experts suggest?

DLB and PDD are the same disease, but have different origins, sharing many of the same symptoms, but the occurrence is different. To distinguish between the diseases, the physicians must perform a cognitive assessment.

Cognitive decline is systematic of both PDD and DLB but does not develop the same. DLB causes erratic levels of cognitive ability, whereas PDD produces a steadier cognitive decline. Thus, the cognitive ability of DLB patients shows drastic improvement in one test, only to decline the next.

Dementia with Lewy bodies begins as dementia and develops Parkinson's disease, while Parkinson's with Lewy bodies begins as Parkinson's disease before developing dementia.

To determine if somebody is suffering PDD or DLB, physicians base their hypothesis on how patients answer questions. The patient and family should document the symptoms in a medical journal and must provide a complete report of symptoms. You never know when such a medical journal might save your life, or at least prolong the quality. Provide your doctor with full access.

And express the full truth when the doctor asks questions.

Once asking questions about symptoms, doctors should conduct a cognitive assessment.

How else do medical experts distinguish between PDD and DLB?

From a clinical standpoint, once the diseases advance, PDD and DLB are the same disease[59]. If Parkinson's disease preceded dementia, it is PDD. If dementia preceded Parkinson's disease, it is DLB. Thus, the diagnosis depends on which disease occurred first.

Experts admit the peculiar distinction, two paths to the same combination of Parkinson's disease, and Lewy body dementia. However, if we've learned anything from dementia research, it is there are many more types or subtypes than we ever imagine.

In this book, we focus on dementia with Lewy bodies (DLB). Let's begin by defining the neurological disorder.

Chapter 6: WHAT IS DEMENTIA WITH LEWY BODIES (DLB)?

People with DLB have a buildup of abnormal protein particles in their brain tissue, called Lewy bodies. Lewy bodies are also found in the brain tissue of people with Parkinson's disease (PD) and Alzheimer's disease (AD). However, in these conditions, the Lewy bodies are generally found in different parts of the brain.

The presence of Lewy bodies in DLB, PD, and AD suggests a connection among these conditions. But scientists haven't yet figured out what the connection is.

DLB affects a person's ability to think, reason, and process information. It can also affect movement, personality, and memory

–Cedars-Sinal[60]

Some suggest dementia with Lewy bodies and Lewy body dementia are the same. Yes and no.

As already covered, dementia with Lewy bodies and Parkinson's disease dementia become Lewy body dementia, so the question is whether they start Lewy body dementia or evolve. Researchers cannot yet answer the question.

Also, if Dementia with Lewy bodies and Lewy body dementia are the same, by the same logic, so would be Parkinson's disease dementia. For this book, dementia with Lewy bodies and Parkinson's disease dementia are two branches of Lewy body dementia.

Alzheimer's Association describes dementia with Lewy bodies[61]:

Dementia with Lewy bodies (DLB) is a progressive dementia that leads to a decline in thinking, reasoning, and independent function because of abnormal microscopic deposits that damage brain cells over time.

How prevalent is dementia with Lewy bodies?

According to the Lewy Body Dementia Association (LBDA), Lewy bodies are the second most prevalent form of dementia[62]. The LBDA claims dementia with Lewy bodies is the most misdiagnosed and underdiagnosed of all dementias[63].

View the cortex and spinal stem in the image.

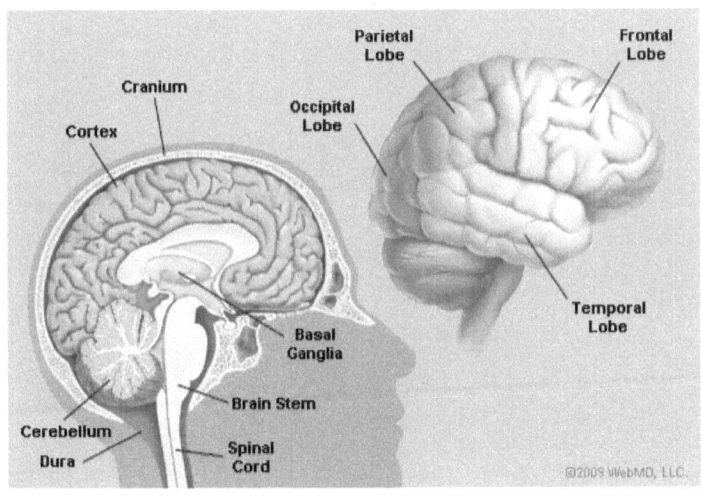

Brain Parts[64]

Dementia with Lewy bodies is the second or third most common dementia, accounting for 10 to 25 percent of dementia occurrence. Since the number of dementia with Lewy bodies and vascular dementia are estimates, not actual, the ranking depends if the real numbers are on the low or high end.

Chapter 7: WHAT IS PARKINSON'S DISEASE? (PD)

The medical community named Parkinson's disease (PD) after Dr. James Parkinson, the British physician who discovered the disease in 1817 and described it in *An Essay on the Shaking Palsy*.

The second most prevalent neurodegenerative disorder, behind Alzheimer's, Parkinson's disease (PD), strikes more people than "multiple sclerosis (MS), muscular dystrophy (MD), and amyotrophic lateral sclerosis (ALS) combined[65]."

Let's turn to Parkinson's authorities to see how they define the disease.

According to the Parkinson's Foundation, Parkinson's disease is a "neurodegenerative disorder that affects predominately dopamine-producing (dopaminergic) neurons in a specific area of the brain called the substantia nigra[66]."

Now, let's view a Parkinson's description in everyday language.

The American Parkinson Disease Association describes Parkinson's disease.

> *Parkinson's disease is a type of movement disorder that can affect the ability to perform common, daily activities. It is a chronic and progressive disease, meaning that the symptoms become worse over time. It is characterized by its most common of motor symptoms – tremors (a form of rhythmic shaking), stiffness or rigidity of the muscles, and slowness of movement (called bradykinesia) – but also manifests in non-motor symptoms including sleep problems, constipation, anxiety, depression, and fatigue, among others[67].*

How many people have Parkinson's disease?

One million Americans and over 10 million people worldwide live with Parkinson's disease[68].

Is Parkinson's disease hereditary?

Genetics causes less than ten percent, although scientists have yet to identify the cause for the other 90 percent of Parkinson's cases. Researchers figured out what happens once Parkinson's disease manifests, but not why.

Who does Parkinson's disease strike?

Whereas women are more likely to get most dementias than men, men are 1.5 times more likely than women to get Parkinson's disease. Although more prevalent among black women, Parkinson's attacks women less than men.

Who are the three highest risk groups?

Highest PDD Risk Groups

- Males
- Hispanics
- Whites

What percentage of Parkinson's disease develops dementia?

Researchers calculate 50-80 percent of Parkinson's disease (PD) develop dementia[69]. Once diagnosed, their status becomes Parkinson's disease dementia (PDD).

What is Parkinson's disease dementia (PDD)?

When Parkinson's disease develops dementia symptoms, the medical profession calls it Parkinson's disease dementia

(PDD).

Chapter 8: WHAT IS CORTICOBASAL SYNDROME (CBS)?

Another FTD disorder, the first official report of corticobasal syndrome (CBS), was in 1967 when Jean J. Rebeiz and colleague documented three patients with slow, clumsy movements that grew progressively worse[70].

Rebeiz and others continued to study the mysterious disorder for two more decades before WR Gibb and colleagues developed the name to corticobasal degeneration and provided an abbreviation (CBD) for a second distinction[71].

Also called CBS attacks the brain's frontal and temporal lobes.

To help form an image of CBS, the Baylor College of Medicine describes CBS as "a Parkinsonism-plus syndrome.

Atypical parkinsonism, Corticobasal syndrome (CBS) attacks the brain's cerebral cortical and basal ganglia regions, which play significant roles in the motor movement. CBS causes problems with balance, muscle control, memory, and speech[72].

Although CBS shares some but not all Parkinson's symptoms, they are two different disorders. Besides different symptoms, CBS does not respond to the same to treatment as Parkinson's.

According to the Journal of Neuropsychiatry[73]:

> CBD is a neurodegenerative dementia with abnormal movements and focal behavioral manifestations. The clinical diagnosis is difficult to make in the absence of pathological findings. Functional imaging studies may be very helpful in demonstrating asymmetrical abnormalities in frontoparietal regions, basal ganglia, and

thalamus contralateral to clinical symptoms,
particularly in the early stages.

What is the Difference between Corticobasal syndrome (CBS) and Corticobasal Degeneration (CBD)?

One glaring difference between CBS and CBD is their sometimes divergent pathologies. A specific tauopathy leads to corticobasal degeneration (CBD), but Alzheimer's sometimes explains corticobasal syndrome (CBS).

CBS Prevalence

According to NORD, CBS attacks five of every 100,000 people[74].

Who Gets CBS?

Most studies suggest CBS assaults men and women in near equal numbers, although a few suggest women are at a slightly higher risk.

Although there are documented cases of corticobasal syndrome striking people as young as 28, CBS strikes people age 50-70 most the time.

CBS Life Expectancy

From the time symptoms manifest, the average life expectancy is eight years. However, some do not make it for eight years, and others have survived up to 17 years.

What Causes CBS?

Like many dementias, scientists remain baffled about what causes corticobasal syndrome (CBS).

We know there is tau protein buildup associated with some CBS patients, while others exhibit the amyloid protein associated with Alzheimer's. However, we do not know why the protein turns rogue[75].

If this story sounds familiar, it's the same old song with several dementias.

One reason we have not developed a cure for CBS, Alzheimer's, and other dementias is that we go about it wrong. Drug studies focus on reducing the dementia-related protein deposits, but this is—at best—the equivalent of chopping a weed above the surface and fails to treat the underlying problem.

In part, it might also explain why each drug trial costs billions of dollars.

II. LEWY BODY & PARKINSONISM DEMENTIAS' SYMPTOMS

This section focuses on symptoms for:
1. *Dementia with Lewy bodies*
2. *Parkinson's disease dementia*
3. Corticobasal syndrome

Each type shares similar symptoms, but also differ. As we discuss in the stages section, DLB, PDD, and CBS also differ in how the symptoms manifest.

Chapter 9: DEMENTIA WITH LEWY BODIES SYMPTOMS

When discussing symptoms for the two primary Lewy body dementias, one must remember the two end up with the same symptoms.

Whereas Parkinson's disease dementia begins with Parkinson's and evolves into dementia, dementia with Lewy bodies starts as dementia and develops Parkinson's disease in later stages. Where the two versions cross paths and become one mystifies science.

With that stipulation, let's examine dementia with Lewy body symptoms.

> *In this gait, the patient will have rigidity and bradykinesia. He or she will be stooped with the head and neck forward, with flexion at the knees. The whole upper extremity is also in flexion, with the fingers usually extended. The patient walks with slow little steps known as Marche a petits pas (walk of little steps). {The} Patient may also have difficulty initiating steps. The patient may show an involuntary inclination to take accelerating steps, known as festination. This gait is seen in Parkinson's disease or any other condition causing parkinsonism, such as side effects from drugs.*

> *–Stanford Medicine*[76]

What are the symptoms of dementia with Lewy bodies?

Dementia with Lewy Bodies Symptoms

We break dementia with Lewy bodies' symptoms into five categories: behavioral and mood, cognitive, movement problems, sleep, and others.

The list below outlines dementia with Lewy bodies' symptoms.

Behavioral And Mood Symptoms

People who have dementia with Lewy bodies experience six primary behavioral and mood symptoms.

- Agitation
- Apathy
- Anxiety
- Delusions
- Depression
- Paranoia

Cognitive Symptoms

DLB cognitive symptoms include cognitive fluctuations and dementia. Expect changes in personality, thinking, and reasoning[77]. DLB patients experience confusion, often occurring off and on[78]. DLB produces delusions[79], hallucinations[80], and memory issues that might fluctuate at different parts of the day[81]. Patients often appear unmotivated[82].

Motor Symptoms

Those suffering DLB suffer a variety of movement problems. DLB patients move slow, unsteady, unsure[83]. As the disease progresses, it causes Parkinson's symptoms, including balance issues, hunching[84]. DLB sufferers also experience problems judging distance[85].

DLB Movement Problems Symptoms include:

- Balance disorder[86]
- Coordination decline

- Blank facial expressions[87]
- Falling[88]
- Muscle rigidity
- Muscle stiffness
- Shaking while resting
- Shuffled walk
- Stooped posture
- Swallowing problems
- Tremor
- Speaking problems[89]
- Writing becomes smaller

Sleep Symptoms

DLB causes daytime sleepiness, insomnia, REM sleep behavior disorder (RBD), and restless leg syndrome.

Sleep disorders connected to DLB include violent outbursts while suffering uncomfortable dreams[90].

Other Symptoms

DLB patients also suffer choking[91] and fainting[92], problems with blood pressure and body temperature, urinary incontinence, and sexual dysfunction. Other symptoms include chest infections[93], constipation, and a diminished sense of smell.

Other DLB Sources: Mayo Clinic[94], National Institute on Aging (NIH)[95], Lewy Body Dementia Association[96], National Health Services (NHS)[97]

Chapter 10: PARKINSON'S DISEASE DEMENTIA (PDD) SYMPTOMS

In this gait, the patient will have rigidity and bradykinesia. He or she will be stooped with the head and neck forward, with flexion at the knees. The whole upper extremity is also in flexion, with the fingers usually extended. The patient walks with slow little steps known as Marche a petits pas (walk of little steps). {The} patient may also have difficulty initiating steps. The patient may show an involuntary inclination to take accelerating steps, known as festination. This gait is seen in Parkinson's disease or any other condition causing parkinsonism, such as side effects from drugs.

–Stanford Medicine[98]

We divide Parkinson's disease dementia symptoms into two categories, motor, and non-motor.

PDD SYMPTOMS

Motor symptoms

Parkinson's causes a wide variety of motor problems, including balance and gait issues and bradykinesia (slow movements). PDD patients suffer from stiffness, and moving grows more difficult, including walking.

PDD patients' postures stoop. They often suffer tremors (involuntary twitching and movements).

Behavioral And Mood Symptoms

Parkinson's patients suffer a variety of behavioral and mood problems, the most prevalent being anxiety and depression.

According to Anna Morenkova, MD, Ph.D., UCI School of Medicine's Department of Neurology, PDD patients also go through personality changes.

"A person who was always conscientious becomes careless," said Norenkova. "A previously easy-going person becomes rigid and stubborn An outgoing social butterfly turns into a stay-at-home introvert."

Cognitive Issues

Cognitive issues include attention deficits, slower thinking, and decreased executive function. Parkinson's patients often struggle for the correct word. Learning grows progressively more difficult because Parkinson's attacks the part of the brain responsible for remembering. PDD patients also suffer visuospatial dysfunction.

Sleep Symptoms

Parkinson's patients suffer several sleep problems, including REM, vivid nightmares, sleep fragmentation (continuous awakening), and sleep apnea.

The sleep issues compound the other Parkinson's symptoms, adding another layer of discomfort and anxiety.

Motor Symptoms

Most of us have seen people with Parkinsons' disease. Michael J. Fox. Robin Williams. Muhammad Ali. Parkinsons' struck all three famous men. Indeed, most see so many people with Parkinson's; they mistake other disorders for PD that share "Parkinson's-like" symptoms. Most the Parkinson's symptoms we're familiar with are motor skills.

We watched Parkinson's take down one of the greatest athletes ever. A man who stood for work ethic, confidence, courage, toughness, yet words flowed from his tongue like the greatest poets and orators. Muhammad Ali fought the disease like the champ he was, but most of us cringed watching his great body deteriorate until we only saw him in a wheelchair.

PDD motor symptoms

- Bradykinesia
- Gait/Walking problems
- Dystonia
- Rigidity
- Tremors
- Unstable posture

Other Symptoms

- Constipation
- Dizziness or fainting
- Drooling
- Early satiety
- Fatigue
- Increased dandruff
- Lightheadedness
- Losing the sense of smell or taste
- Pain
- Sexual problems
- Urinary urgency, frequency, and incontinence
- Vision problems
- Weight loss

Parkinson's Symptoms Sources: European Parkinson's Disease Association[99], Alzheimer's Society[100], Parkinson's Foundation[101], The Lancet Neurology[102], *Parkinson' News Today*[103], EPDA[104], Parkinson's Foundation[105], LBDA[106]

Chapter 11:
CORTICOBASAL SYNDROME (CBS) SYMPTOMS

Often misdiagnosed for Parkinson's disease, corticobasal syndrome causes a wide range of symptoms affecting speech and language, memory and cognitive skills, movement, and motor skills.

In this chapter, we outline corticobasal syndrome symptoms and then discuss more in the stages section.

Corticobasal Syndrome Symptoms List

- Acalculia
- Akinesia
- Alien limb phenomenon
- Apraxia
- Bradykinesia
- Dystonia
- Visuospatial disorder

The list shows corticobasal syndrome attacking motor and cognitive skills.

Before moving on, let's discuss each symptom. While the subject matter goes beyond this book, I want to provide a brief description for anybody who might not understand or recognize any of the listed disorders.

CBS Symptoms

Acalculia

Perhaps the rarest connection to corticobasal syndrome, acalculia attacks the part of the brain responsible for mathematics[107]. A person who skillfully handled math who develops acalculia might struggle with basic addition, subtraction, multiplication, and division.

Akinesia

One reason people refer to CBS as atypical Parkinsonism is because both disorders cause akinesia. When somebody has akinesia, they cannot make something move.

Somebody suffering akinesia cannot move muscles voluntarily[108]. For instance, akinesia prevents the arms from swinging back and forth, which normally does so without thought. Akinesia also causes other movement problems.

Damaged neurons cannot signal the muscles and nerves to move. Akinesia causes immeasurable frustration for CBS, Parkinson's, stroke, and other neurological disorders.

Alien Limb Phenomenon

The opposite of akinesia, alien limb phenomenon, causes involuntary movement. Also known as Dr. Strangelove's syndrome, alien limb phenomenon is an important CBS diagnosis factor[109].

Patients often feel separated from their limbs, and the movements cause significant stress.

Apraxia

Apraxia is somewhat the opposite of the alien limb phenomenon. When somebody experiences apraxia, they fail to perform learned movements[110]. Aware of what they want to do, the brain no longer follows their commands.

Prominent in Corticobasal syndrome (CBS) is limb apraxia, which causes limited use or paralysis in an arm, hand, or leg.

The American Speech-Language-Hearing Association

describes limb apraxia: "A disorder of motor planning in the absence of impaired muscle control that affects voluntary positioning and sequencing of muscle movements of the limbs[111]."

Stroke patients also suffer apraxia, which is why neurologists sometimes misdiagnose corticobasal syndrome for stroke.

Bradykinesia

Brain damage causes bradykinesia, a disorder causing slow movement.

Bradykinesia resembles akinesia, but they are not synonymous. The *Journal of Neurology* explains the difference:

> *Bradykinesia describes the slowness of a performed movement, whereas akinesia refers to a poverty of spontaneous movement (e.g., in facial expression) or associated movement (e.g., arm swing during walking). Other manifestations of akinesia are freezing, and the prolonged time it takes to initiate a movement[112].*

Bradykinesia makes a person feel as if they are moving in slow motion. Whatever their normal speed, most movements slow. Somebody suffering bradykinesia struggles to tap their finger, tap a foot, or move palms up and down at any speed[113].

Dystonia

Dystonia causes uncontrollable muscle contractions in certain parts or the entire body.

According to the Dystonia Medical Research Foundation: "Dystonia can affect any region of the body including the eyelids, face, jaw, neck, vocal cords, torso, limbs, hands, and feet. Depending on the region of the body affected, dystonia may look quite different from person to person[114]." Dystonia Medical warns dystonia causes enormous anxiety and severe depression.

The American Association of Neurological Surgeons

explains dystonia's complexity.

> *Dystonia is a very complex, highly variable*
> *neurological movement disorder characterized by*
> *involuntary muscle contractions. As many as*
> *250,000 people in the United States have*
> *dystonia, making it the third most common*
> *movement disorder behind essential tremor and*
> *Parkinson's disease*[115].

Parkinson's-like symptoms such as dystonia are why most consider corticobasal syndrome a Parkinsonism-plus disorder.

Visuospatial Disorder

Our visuospatial network helps create our unique vantage point.

Normal visual-spatial processing establishes our presence or place in the world compared to the space, objects, animals, and people around us.

Visuospatial disorder destroys the ability to make sense of objects, animals, and people surrounding us. Somebody suffering a visuospatial disorder cannot find things a few feet away, including the bathroom or familiar objects[116].

The problem is not the eyes, which might be perfect, but our brain's ability to process, establish, and maintain our place in the world.

Visuospatial disorders make it difficult or impossible for one to determine distance. The breakdowns cause mass confusion and make it difficult for somebody to find something feet away from such as stairs (not recommended for somebody suffering a visuospatial disorder) or the bathroom.

A severe visuospatial disorder places a person in a perpetual state of disorientation.

Chapter 12: LEWY BODY-PARKINSONISM DEMENTIA SYMPTOMS RECAP

Dementias share several similarities, complicating diagnosis. Each dementia category recap includes compilation tables dividing and comparing specific symptom types to help diagnosis.

- Cognitive
- Psychological (including emotional and behavior)
- Motor
- Language
- Visual/Perception

The tables help doctors and patients narrow down the possibilities when diagnosing the 19 primary dementias accounting for 99% of dementia.

Lewy Body/Parkinsonism Cognitive Symptoms

COGNITIVE SYMPTOM	DLB	PDD	CBS
Attention-deficit		X	
Cognitive fluctuations	X		
Executive skills decline		X	
Hallucinations	X		
Learning disability		X	
Paranoia	X		
Memory fluctuations	X	X	
Personality changes	X	X	
Reasoning decline	X		
Thinking decline	X	X	
Unmotivated	X		
Visuospatial dysfunction		X	X

DLB = dementia with lewy bodies

PDD = Parkinson's disease dementia

CBS = Corticobasal syndrome

DLB and PDD both exhibit far more cognitive symptoms than CBS in the diagnosis stage. Although DLB and PDD both cause several cognitive problems, they are mostly different symptoms.

The cognitive symptom table comparison provides doctors a set of symptoms separating the three subtypes.

Lewy Body/Parkinsonism Psychological Symptoms

PSYCHOLOGICAL SYMPTOM	DLB	PDD	CBS
Agitation	X		
Apathy	X		
Anxiety	X	X	
Delusions	X		
Depression	X	X	

DLB = dementia with lewy bodies

PDD = Parkinson's disease dementia

CBS = Corticobasal syndrome

Since dementia with Lewy bodies (DLB) begins with dementia, DLB causes far more behavior and mood problems than PDD or CBS.

Lewy Body/Parkinsonism Motor Symptoms

MOTOR SKILLS SYMPTOM	DLB	PDD	CBS
Acalculia			X
Akinesia		X	X
Alien limb phenomenon			X
Apraxia			X
Balance disorder	X		
Blank facial expressions	X		
Bradykinesia		X	X
Coordination decline	X		
Dystonia		X	X
Falling	X		
Gait/Walking problems		X	
Muscle rigidity	X	X	
Muscle stiffness	X		
Shaking while resting	X		
Shuffled walk	X		
Stooped posture	X		
Swallowing problems	X		
Tremor	X	X	
Speaking problems	X		
Smaller handwriting	X		
Unstable posture		X	
Visuospatial disorder		X	X

DLB = dementia with lewy bodies

PDD = Parkinson's disease dementia

CBS = Corticobasal syndrome

All three subtypes suffer several motor skill disorders. Early-stage Parkinson's symptoms resemble corticobasal syndrome (CBS) far more than dementia with Lewy bodies (DLB).

Although sharing several symptoms with PDD, corticobasal syndrome (CBS) distinguishes itself by having almost entirely motor skill disorders. Doctors rule out CBS when the nonmotor symptoms better fit the PDD pathology.

Lewy Body/Parkinsonism Sleep Symptoms

SLEEP SYMPTOM	DLB	PDD	CBS
Daytime sleepiness	X		
Inability to remain asleep		X	
Insomnia	X		
REM sleep behavior disorder	X		
Responds violently to dreams	X		

DLB = dementia with lewy bodies

PDD = Parkinson's disease dementia

CBS = Corticobasal syndrome

DLB, PDD, and CBS all develop some sleeping problems in late stages but is most prominent in dementia with Lewy bodies (DLB).

DLB patients suffer most every sleep problem imaginable, while Parkinson's patients have more problems staying asleep.

Side effects of medication can cause vivid dreams and nightmares in all three subtypes.

Lewy Body/Parkinsonism Language Symptoms

LANGUAGE SYMPTOMS	DLB	PDD	CBS
Correct word trouble		X	

While Parkinson's disease dementia (PDD), and Corticobasal syndrome (CBS), and dementia with Lewy bodies develop dementia-related language problems in late stages, they do not suffer language problems in the early stages like the primary progressive aphasias. However, PDD patients often struggle to find the correct word.

Lewy Body/Parkinsonism Other Symptoms

OTHER SYMPTOMS	DLB	PDD	CBS
Reduced blinking (leads to dry eyes)		X	
Blood pressure problems	X		
Body temperature issues	X		
Chest infections	X		
Choking	X		
Constipation	X	X	
A diminished sense of smell	X		
Dizziness		X	
Drooling		X	
Early satiety		X	
Excessive perspiration		X	
Fainting	X	X	
Fatigue		X	
Increased dandruff		X	
Lightheadedness		X	
Pain		X	
Sense of smell loss		X	
Sexual dysfunction	X		
Urinary discomfort & urgency		X	
Urinary incontinence	X	X	
Vision problems		X	
Weight loss		X	

DLB = dementia with lewy bodies

PDD = Parkinson's disease dementia

CBS = Corticobasal syndrome

    The tables show dementia with Lewy bodies (DLB, Parkinson's disease dementia (PDD), and corticobasal syndrome (CBS) share many symptoms, especially motor skill decline.

    However, the charts also show divergence, which is crucial in making the correct diagnosis. While PDD and DLB turn into the same dementia, they take opposite routes. PDD begins with Parkinson's and develops dementia years later, whereas DLB begins with dementia and develops Parkinson's later.

    The only reason they are not one disorder is because of their divergent pathologies.

    Corticobasal syndrome shares some characteristics with DLB and especially PDD, but does not evolve into the same disorder as DLB and PDD.

Lewy body/Parkinsonism Symptoms

To this point, we outlined the symptoms for each dementia. Let's discuss some primary symptoms in greater detail.

Blank facial expressions

Somebody with dementia with Lewy Bodies or Parkinson's disease cannot express certain emotions through facial expressions.

The Lewy Body Dementia Association lists blank facial expressions as a symptom for both Parkinson's disease and dementia with Lewy bodies[117].

People with either Lewy body dementia often stare into space or has a blank expression[118].

A *PubMed* study of facial expressions of people with Parkinson's disease, Parkinson's disease dementia, or dementia with Lewy bodies found the patients could not identify anger, fear, and sadness.

"There were several facial expressions that the Lewy body disease patients {could not} accurately identify," the study concluded. "Caregivers are recommended to {attempt} to compensate for such situations with language or body contact, etc., to convey the correct feeling to the patients of each type[119]."

Fainting

While fainting suggests many health issues, it is one symptom doctors consider when diagnosing the Lewy body dementias[120].

Parkinson's disease and dementia with Lewy bodies often include a series of injuries caused by fainting.

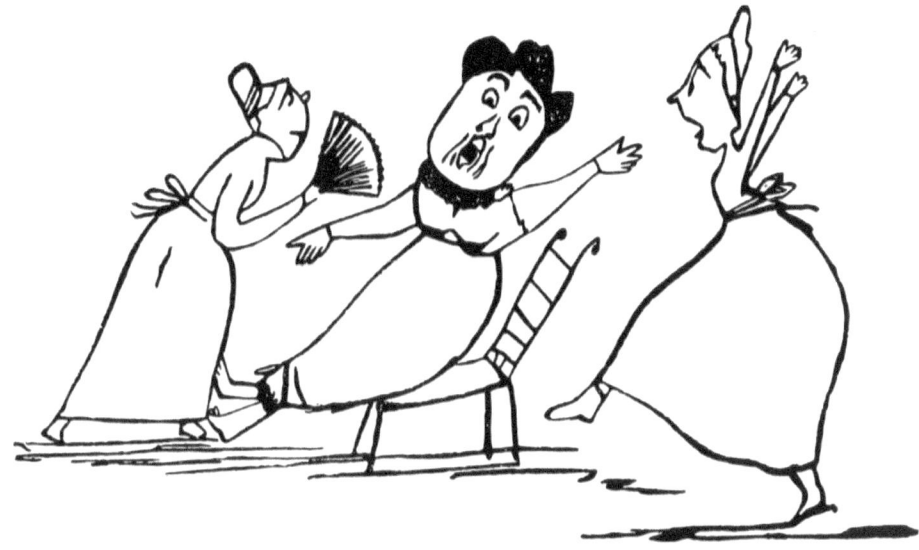

Changes in personality, thinking, and reasoning

When diagnosing either of the Lewy body dementias, doctors check for personality, thinking, and reasoning changes.

A group of researchers from the Washington University School of Medicine in St. Louis studied an equal number of Lewy body dementia and Alzheimer's patients to find a better way of distinguishing the two similar diseases.

The researchers found those with Lewy body dementia were twice as likely as Alzheimer's patients to develop personality changes[121].

"We look for memory problems and other cognitive problems to detect dementia, but personality changes can often occur several years before the cognitive problems," explained lead author James Galvin, M.D. "Identifying the earliest features of dementia may enable doctors to begin therapy as soon as possible. Early diagnosis becomes increasingly important as newer, disease-modifying medications develop. It also gives the patient and family members more time to plan for the progressive decline."

What is the significance?

"Our results show incorporating a brief, simple inventory of personality traits," said Galvin, "may help improve the detection of dementia with Lewy bodies."

Be on the outlook for changes in personality, thinking, and reasoning. The combination might indicate Lewy body dementia.

Chest infections

Chest infections, combined with other symptoms, could suggest one of the Lewy body dementias.

Choking

Choking issues merit medical attention, but combined with other symptoms could implicate Parkinson's disease or dementia with Lewy bodies.

Confusion, often occurring off and on

Lewy body dementia confuses, but not constant. Early-stage, the confusion and coherency switch out on a moment's notice.

In the early stage, a person remains semi-functional. Somebody with DLB goes through stretches where they seem their old self, but the "episodes" grow more frequent and severe.

Shocking, frightening, and bewildering, the moments of confusion shake a person's inner core. At first, one might attribute the bad moments to age or other factors, but it is impossible to fool themselves or others for long. A person swims against the tide in stage one, and the current is too strong and diabolical to defeat for long.

Delusional

The result of defective cholinergic activity, DLB patients, suffer both delusions and hallucinations.

Delusions often center around the strong belief somebody is trying to steal something. DLB patients suffering delusions suffer more significant neuropsychiatric symptoms and greater cognitive decline[122].

Whereas hallucinations do not usually unsettle DLB patients, delusions often upset and cause behavioral problems.

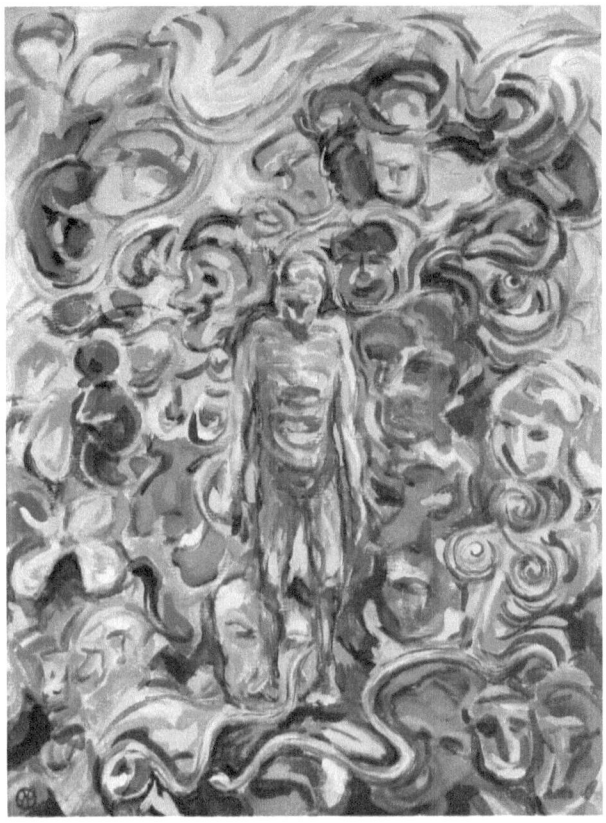

When somebody with DLB accuses somebody of stealing, they do so with absolute conviction. Once upset, a person often says cruel things, but remember it is dementia. Although their behavior might grow belligerent and unacceptable by any normal standards, there is nothing normal about dementia.

Talk them down. Keep a safe distance if the situation poses a danger. Whatever you do, do not argue, do not respond in anger, and do not allow dementia words to hurt your feelings. If they did not feel this way before getting dementia, you must accept they now suffer a fatal disease attacking their cognitive skills.

Treat them like somebody threatening to jump off a high roof. Recognize AD patients are in pain and ease them down.

Falling

Because of delusions, fainting, and balance issues, DLB patients suffer many falls. The injuries grow more severe and frequent as the disease advances. By the end, falls often are the direct cause of death.

Hallucinations

People with Parkinson's disease or dementia with Lewy bodies might suffer hallucinations. According to the Columbia University Department of Neurology, about. 80% of DLB sufferers experience visual hallucinations[123].

While quite vivid, and often unsettling for others, Columbia reports the hallucinations do not typically disturb the patient. Mild symptoms require no medication, but neurologists prescribe acetylcholinesterase inhibitors for more severe cases[124].

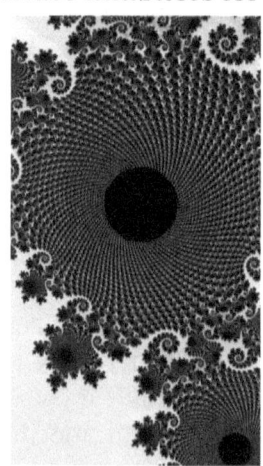

DLB Movement problems. Slow. Unsteady.

Another symptom of Lewy body dementia is slow or unsteady movement issues; one of the many Parkinson's symptoms one develops as DLB progresses.

DLB attacks the part of the brain responsible for coordinating movement, resulting in diminished coordination, balance, and movement.

Physical therapists work with DLB patients to help restore balance and movement where possible and to slow digression. I consider physical therapists pivotal in treating Parkinson's related neurological disorders.

Like speech therapists (and other types), physical therapists often help stroke and dementia patients retrain the brain to regain mobility, speech, and other handicaps. Therapists help prolong one's quality of life, perhaps the greatest gift for somebody diagnosed with dementia.

III. LEWY BODY DEMENTIA/PARKINSONISM STAGES

Having covered and compared symptoms for dementia with Lewy bodies, Parkinson's disease dementia, and corticobasal syndrome, let's view how they play out through stages.

Chapter 13: DEMENTIA WITH LEWY BODIES STAGES

This chapter focuses on DLB stages. Unlike Parkinson's disease dementia (PDD), dementia with Lewy bodies, early-stage symptoms include cognitive deterioration.

Another distinguishing DLB characteristic is a wild fluctuation in attention, almost normal one day, then serious the next, or from morning to afternoon[125].

Dementia with Lewy Bodies Early Stages

Often within a year, dementia with Lewy bodies develops symptoms similar to Alzheimer's, on the one hand, and other symptoms resembling Parkinson's disease.

Despite the similarities, DLB differs from Alzheimer's in many ways. Whereas in early stages, Alzheimer's tends to attack memory, DLB patients suffer much fewer initial memory issues. Also, in the early stages, behavioral issues are a bigger issue for DLB than Alzheimer's patients.

DLB Stage 1

During stage one dementia with Lewy bodies, symptoms alarm both the person who is experiencing the symptoms and their loved ones and close associates.

In stage one, a person might remain independent in socialization, but experience difficulty driving.

Stage one symptoms include:

Behavioral And Mood

Stage one behavioral and mood symptoms include anxiety, depression, and erratic mood swings.

Cognitive

Since dementia with Lewy bodies begins as dementia and progresses to Parkinsonism, LBD produces several stage one cognitive symptoms.

- Atypical difficulty handling finances or planning
- Atypical pronunciation problems
- Declining comprehension
- Declining executive skills
- Difficulty learning new tasks
- Difficulty selecting the correct word
- Deteriorating handwriting skills
- Diminished hearing
- A diminished sense of smell
- Hallucinations
- Paranoia
- Peripheral deterioration
- Problem-solving impairment
- An impaired short term memory
- Unmotivated
- Vision impairment

Movement Problems

Stage one DLB causes jerky movements, reduced coordination, shuffling gait, and other Parkinson's related symptoms. Early manifestations include slower movements and stooping or leaning posture. In stage one, these symptoms are less pronounced than the dementia-related symptoms but grow progressively worse.

Sleep

DLB produces a variety of sleep problems, including REM sleep disorder and restless leg syndrome. Dementia with Lewy bodies also makes people sleep two or more hours during the day.

Other

- Continuous runny nose

In the latter half of stage one, the number and severity of symptoms make seeing a doctor obvious. Something is wrong!

DLB Stage 2

Although suffering several symptoms from the stage 1 list, doctors often misdiagnose DLB for Alzheimer's disease, Parkinson's disease, or multisystem atrophy.

Although the correct diagnosis is a longshot, it is important by now to establish a Power of Attorney for general and medical power to make difficult decisions.

Patients and loved ones must make several important financial decisions during this period.

The stage two symptoms include those listed for stage one, plus:

Behavioral And Mood

Stage one behavioral and mood problems grow more severe in stage two. Agitation and depression worsen.

Cognitive

Besides stage one cognitive issues becoming more burdensome, stage two symptoms include:

- Aphasia-related difficulty finding words
- Delusions worsen
- Further concentration decline
- Reading ability declines
- Scattered thoughts

Movement Problems

Stage one movement problems worsen in stage two. A person experiences more difficulty balancing, and falling becomes a greater problem, both in volume and severity. Parkinson's symptoms grow more pronounced.

Sleep

REM sleep disorder and restless leg syndrome problems worsen in stage two. A person wants to sleep more and more during the day but experiences greater problems sleeping at night.

Other

- Blood pressure fluctuation
- Capgras syndrome
- Dry mouth
- Fainting
- Incontinence (couple times per month)
- Unusual perspiration

A person might require a walker because of falls but can still move without help. They perform most daily duties, although some are becoming more difficult. They might administer their medication, but I recommend supervision. Following most conversations remains possible, although more difficult.

While 24/7 care is not yet necessary, as stage two develops, the patient requires more supervision and help to perform daily activities.

DLB Stage 3

Symptoms grow more apparent by stage three, making diagnosis easier. Whereas early symptoms often are mistaken for Alzheimer's, by now, clear differences emerge, such as fluctuating mood swings.

A stage three DLB patient now requires assistance with many daily functions, including administering medication.

Stage three symptoms include symptoms from stages one and two, plus:

Behavioral And Mood

All previous behavioral and mood problems worsen. DLB patients suffer severe anxiousness in stage three. Easily angered and often depressed, coping grows more difficult.

Psychological disorders create health risks for patients and caregivers, making caring for loved ones much more difficult.

Home health aide assistance might become necessary.

Cognitive

Stage three cognitive symptoms worsen. DLB patients suffer great confusion during this period. If a person drove or worked in stages one and two, they no longer can do either. The ability to speak continues to decline. A person who suffers tremendous paranoia and mood swings become unbearable.

Movement Problems

Ambulation declines, and the autonomic dysfunctions (mild to fatal). Whereas the cognitive and behavioral issues were more problematic in stages one and two, Parkinsonism symptom grow more pronounced in stage three, and the risk of falls heighten.

Sleep

Sleeping problems worsen. For many or most, getting a quality night's sleep grows near impossible. Sleepy during the day and unable to sleep at night too often become routine.

Other

Incontinence incidents increase in stage three. More problematic, many DLB patients suffer heat transfer deterioration, preventing the movement of heat to fluids.

Good moments become rarer during stage three, so families must enjoy each as if they might be the last. Hopefully, there are more to come, but the DLB patient's body and mind are losing the battle. Not only is the end near, but the quality of life diminishes.

DLB Stage 4

Stage three brought more severe symptoms, but everything worsens in stage four. If the loved one does not already have 24/7 supervision, they require it now.

Stage four symptoms include all previous listed, plus:

Behavioral And Mood

Many are in a continuous cycle of depression and anxiety. These and other tormenting emotions burn within DLB patients in stage four.

While they cannot verbalize their thoughts as often or clear, they suffer no less inner turmoil.

Cognitive

Speaking becomes more challenging. The world makes less sense, and, as aphasia worsens, articulating thoughts becomes much more difficult.

Movement Problems

Parkinson's works with dementia during stage four to devastate a human being. A person requires help with all daily functions, including eating and going to the bathroom.

Drooling is a prominent stage four symptom, but that's the least of problems. All of Parkinson's symptoms worsen.

Sleep

If a person could, they would choose to sleep 24/7 at this point. Of course, the sleep issues prevent them from getting a good night's sleep, so sleeping away their agony is not an option.

Other

- Autonomic dysfunctions
- Incontinence issues heighten
- Needs ambulation help
- Needs transfer assistance
- Requires help with daily activities
- Severe swallowing problems

In stages one through three, the DLB patient and family accepted fate and crossed a difficult valley. Instead of bringing relief, stage four was like putting everything you have to cross the wicked valley, only to find something much worse.

But, stage four is only the prelude for something much worse.

DLB Stage 5

Although some survive for two decades, according to UCSF Weill Institute for Neuroscience[126], the average life span once diagnosed with dementia with Lewy bodies is five to seven years[127].

Somebody in late-stage dementia with Lewy bodies requires 24/7 care.

Stage five is the last waltz. Parties must honor the Living Will.

Families and medical authorities summon hospice or equivalent. Family and friends should also step in when possible to relieve the voluntary caregiver, for they are likely suffering depression, anxiety, fatigue, and the sense of being overwhelmed.

If the patient remains home, they require a hospital bed.

Stage five symptoms include stage one-four symptoms, plus:

Behavioral And Mood

Speaking is difficult, movement limited, and the cognitive decline severe, so a person is not capable of the earlier displays of outrage, but they still suffer. How could they not?

In stage five, a person lives in a perpetual state of delusion. Depressed, anxious, and filled with confusion, pain, and agony, they hurt more physically and emotionally than the rest of us can imagine, even when seeing it firsthand.

Cognitive

If one's language skills survived stage four, they lose them now, maintaining minimum or none. Their comprehension and attention span becomes limited.

Movement Problems

The distinction between dementia with Lewy bodies (DLB) and Parkinson's disease dementia (PDD) becomes impossible during stage four. Parkinson's symptoms turn critical for both classifications during stage five.

Choking becomes routine, and swallowing issues cause malnutrition.

Parkinson's destroys the body. Rigidity becomes critical, and the swallowing issues necessitate a feeding tube. Muscle contractions also become a greater burden, and their bodies and head lean during stage five.

Sleep

Sleep is dear during stage five. Restless and behind on sleep, some sleep more during the day by this point than at night.

Other

A weakened immune system increases risks for infections, fever, and pneumonia. Stage five causes skin deterioration and makes a person hypersensitive to touch.

The patient requires help with all daily functions. Necessary equipment includes a suction machine and a Hoyer lift.

Swallowing difficulties make nutritional supplements and drinks necessary. At some point, responsible parties must decide if medical authorities install a feeding tube.

Present science provides no miraculous recovery, making stage five the final act. Pneumonia or other infections are likely causes of death.

We can only hope the loved one lived a worthy life, one full of more joys than sorrow, and wish them off; however, our spiritual beliefs prompt.

The family and friends should pay attention to the caregiver who too often suffers health problems from years of providing care to a loved one.

The family and loved ones must provide comfort for the dear one suffering DLB and support for the primary caregiver down the stretch. The final months, weeks, and days will challenge your individual and family's inner core.

Remember, you and the family must go on. Let the DLB sufferer go. They've suffered enough, and extending a tormenting life without a cure would be cruel. Take solace knowing they no longer suffer.

Love, cherish, and keep them alive in your memories, but you must learn to live without them. You must find a path to personal fulfillment and happiness. You cannot add to the tragedy by stop living. Honor the fallen by finding a way to thrive!

Stages sources: *Neurology*[128], UCSF Weill Institute for Neuroscience[129], *Oxford Journals*[130], Mayo Clinic[131], Dementia Lewy Bodies Canada[132], Alzheimer's Research & Therapy[133], Lewy Body Support Group[134], Karger[135], American College of Neuropsychopharmacology[136], Udall Parkinson's Disease Center[137], *Journal of Movement Disorders*[138]

Stages Note

Modern medicine keeps DLB and PDD patients alive through stage five, but with no possible cure and to live a torturous and brutalizing last stretch.

Because conventional wisdom has failed to develop a test, vaccine, or cure for DLB and most dementias, we must turn conventional wisdom on its head. Conventional wisdom has led us around the same circle for decades, including failed drug trials, and the more we learn, the more we know we know too little.

I am not encouraging "crackpots," but we must fund independent research that looks outside the box, or at least intends to expand the box.

Having researched and written books on all 19 primary dementia types, I always reach my wit's end by the end of the section on stages. Almost without fail, the dementias share the same ending, cruel and unusual punishment.

For us to win the war against dementia, the governments, corporations, and people with money must invest more in dementia research. That alone, however, will not defeat dementia.

Institutions such as the National Institute on Aging (NIH) who distribute research money must fund respectable and competent neurologists and medical researchers who dare to think outside the box. The current approach is as ineffective in winning the dementia war as the United States Congress has been incompetent and misguided in the Drug War.

If we want to lose the dementia war, we will continue down the same path. If we want to win the dementia war, we must follow trails and beat through the forest's undergrowth to where the answers and solutions reside.

Chapter 14: PARKINSON'S DISEASE DEMENTIA (PDD) STAGES

Parkinson's disease dementia stages manifest as Parkinson's disease. Dementia symptoms might not appear for years.

Parkinson's Disease Stages

Scientists developed several tests over the years to diagnose and monitor Parkinson's disease, but the Unified Parkinson's Disease Rating Scale (UPDRS) combines several and is the most common.

Unified Parkinson's Disease Rating Scale (UPDRS)

Medical professionals presented Unified Parkinson's Disease Rating Scale (UPDRS) in 1987, revised by the Movement Disorder Society (MDS) [139] in 2001 to access non-motor symptoms.

The Unified Parkinson's Disease Rating Scale (UPDRS) is a six-part evaluation, merging several scales and tests to gauge Parkinson's stages.

UPDRS Part One: Mental, Behavior, and Mood Evaluation

This evaluation comes in two stages, part 1A, and part 1B, thirteen total questions[140].

Part 1A

The medical professional will ask thirteen questions concerning non-motor skills. Part 1A focuses on intellectual impairment and thought disorder.

Part 1B

With or without the caregiver's assistance, the patient answers these thirteen questions. It gauges depression, motivation, and initiative.

UPDRS Part Two: Daily Self-Evaluation

Another thirteen questions the patient (and caregiver) answer, but these concern motor skills. There are five grades for each category, ranging from 0 to 4, 0, meaning normal, and 4 showing severest symptoms. Be 100% honest!

Cutting food and handling utensils

If you or a loved one sudden experience difficulty cutting food or handling utensils, this is one warning sign.

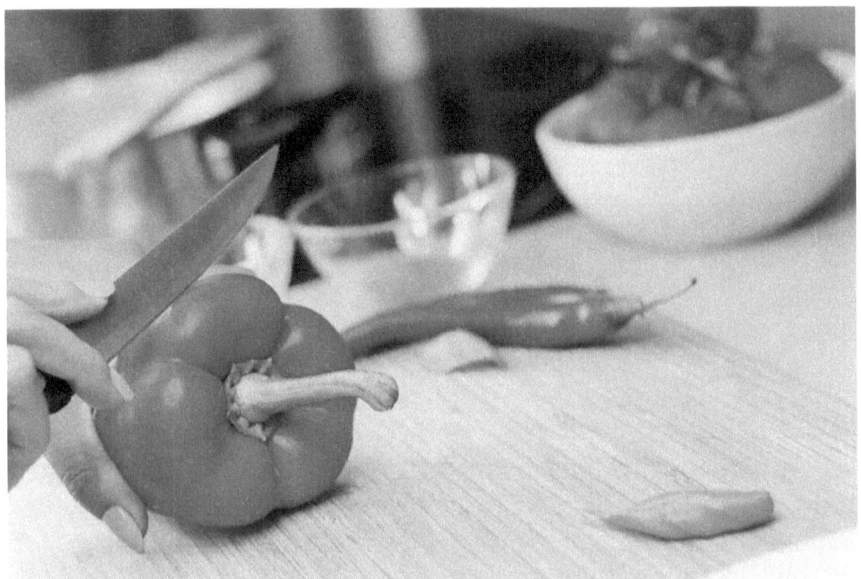

Can you cut, slice, and chop vegetables?

Any issues, slight to serious, report it during this test.

Dressing

If you or loved one experience anything out of the ordinary, such as needing extra help with buttons or zippers, report the severity on this test.

The range is dress as normal, to being helpless by grade four.

Handwriting

The doctor wants to know if you or loved one experience any unusual difficulty handwriting.

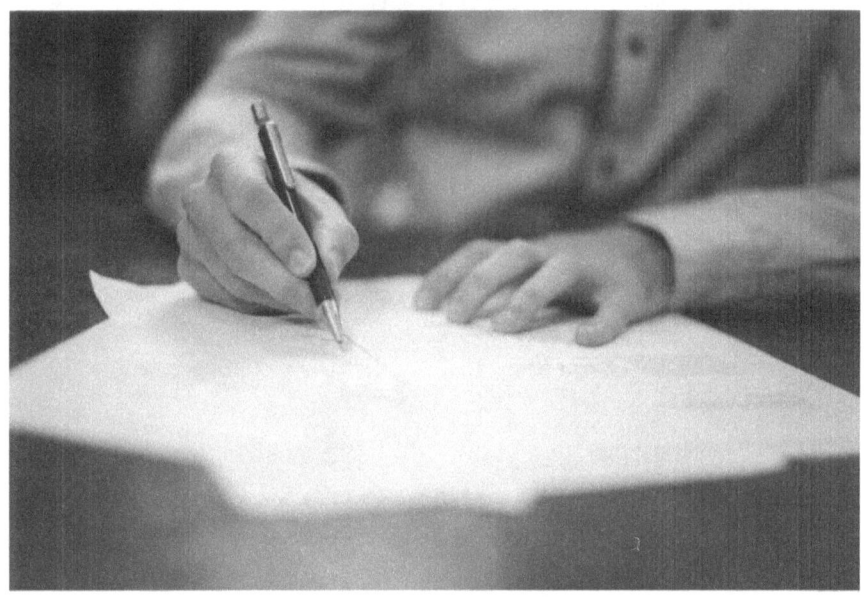

Can you write?

A person with Parkinson's disease writes slow and in letters too small or large. The doctor measures the handwriting's legibility. Often, medical authorities want to see handwriting from years before for comparison.

Hygiene

If hygiene slips, this is another warning sign. Medical officials search for unusual problems. For instance, if somebody flossed their teeth four times a day stops flossing. Or a person who showers three or more times per day stops taking showers.

The activity stands out in both examples more than somebody who normally flosses, brushes their teeth, and showers once a day or less. They designed UPDRS tests to search for such peculiarities.

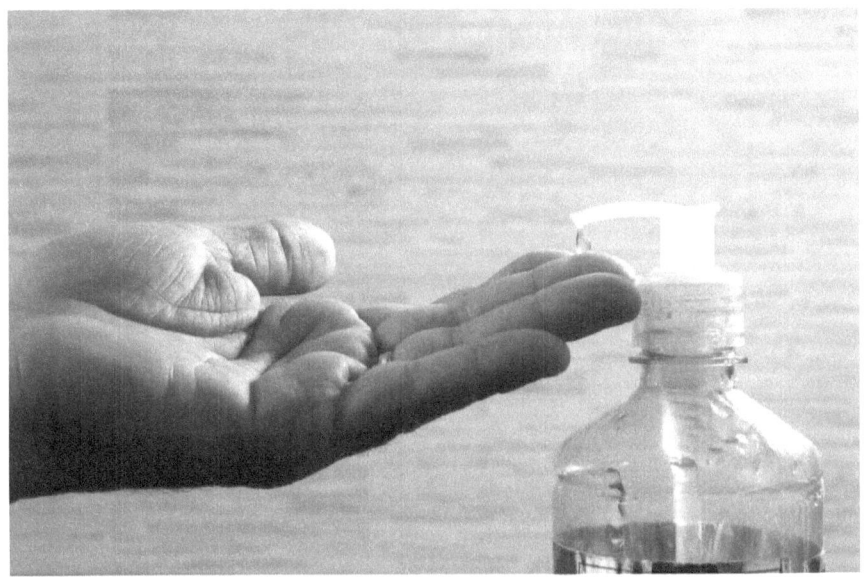

Is hygiene declining?

As with everything, the grades range from 0 to 4, with 0 being normal and 4 meaning extreme decline. Medical officials want to know about any difficulty bathing or other personal hygiene problems. Can the patient:

- Bathe without assistance?
- Brush their teeth?
- Comb their hair?
- Use the bathroom on their own?

To score a grade four, they require a Foley catheter or other medical devices and others to maintain their hygiene.

Falling (unrelated to freezing)

A series of unusual falls will draw caution flags. Doctors also want to know the circumstances leading to the fall(s). Grade one indicates an occasional fall, while a person experiences frequent (almost daily) falls in stage four.

Because it causes injuries, falling is one of the more complicated Parkinsonism symptoms. Protecting them from falls is one of the biggest and most challenging caregiver responsibilities.

Freezing when walking

Freezing makes one feel stuck in place, sometimes leading to falls and accidents. Freezing occurs when walking, sitting, or standing.

An occasional freeze is grade one. Freezing causes frequent falls in stage four.

Salivation

Salivation ranges from excess saliva in the mouth to uncontrollable drooling. A slight problem earns a grade one, and significant problems a grade four.

Like other UPDRS questions, knowing salivation severity helps doctors gauge current PDD advancement.

Speech

Parkinson's disease dementia often causes speech problems, especially as the disease develops. As dementia worsens, so does speech issues in most patients.

The speech grade ranges from 0, normal, to four, unintelligible.

Swallowing

A grade one means infrequent choking, but becomes so frequent by four, they require an NG tube or gastrostomy feeding.

Swallowing issues often cause malnutrition and other related problems.

Tremor

In grade one, a person experiences infrequent and mild tremors. By grade four, the tremors interfere with daily life.

Turning in bed and adjusting bedclothes

Moves "clumsy," but no need for alarm in grade one. By grade four, they are helpless and cannot move.

Parkinson's related sensory complaints

Walking

Walking is one of our greatest gifts, but underutilized. Parkinsonism robs the ability or adds a dangerous element to the otherwise healthy activity.

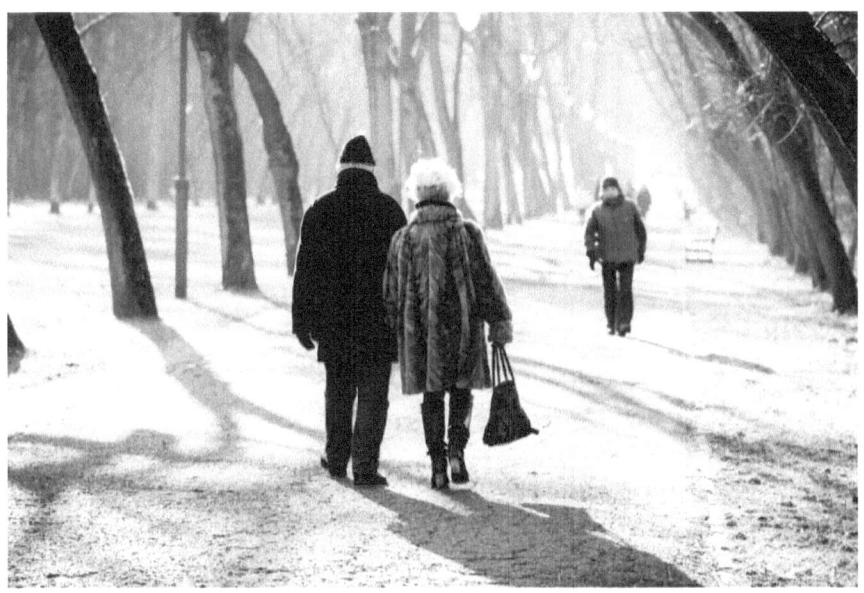

Do you find walking unusually difficult?

With Parkinson's, doctors want to know if you experience any unusual difficulties walking. Doctors measure difficulty in this test to help determine how far the disease has advanced and to address the symptoms.

Grade one means mild difficulty, and four means a person cannot walk, on their own, or assisted.

UPDRS Part Three: Motor Function Evaluation

Part three is a motor function test with 33 scores based on 18 questions.

Action or postural tremor of hands

Grade 1 shows mild tremors of hands in action. By grade four, the patient's tremors grow too severe to feed themselves.

Body Bradykinesia and Hypnokinesis

This segment tests arm swing to determine slow, or diminished amplitude.

In grade one, a person shows mild slowing, and by grade four shows diminished movement amplitude and arm swings.

Facial expression

If a picture is worth a thousand words, facial expressions merit ten thousand.

Most of us visualize a person by their smile or frown, but we make dozens of faces to express our diverse moods and feelings.

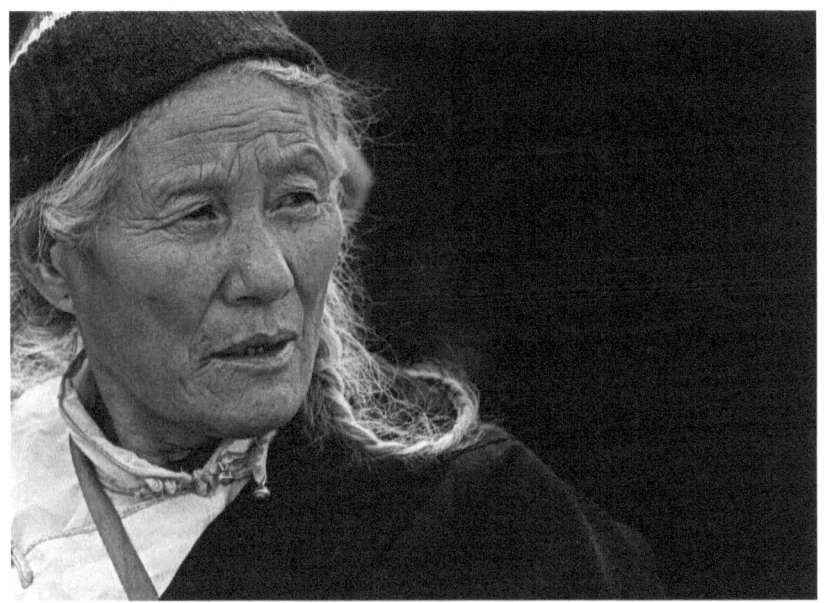

Do you experience hypomimia?

In the grading system, 0 means normal facial expressions, while grade one shows a slight deterioration, but could be a "poker face." Grades two and three indicate an obvious decline, and four show unyielding or veiled expressions, and the mouth opens a quarter-inch or more, and the person experiences near or total hypomimia (loss of facial expression).

Finger taps

In this test, people tap their thumb with their index finger. People show slight difficulty or slowness in grade one while they struggle to touch their thumb by stage four.

Gait

This segment of the test measures one's manner of walking.

Hand movements

Doctors measure how rapid a patient can open and close hands. Grade one means a slight problem where the person slows. By grade four, people struggle to open and close their hands even once.

Leg agility

A person must raise their foot at least three inches and tap heel. To slow or lose amplitude is level one while achieving the exercise becomes near impossible by stage four.

Postural stability

Next, they test postural stability while a person is standing with eyes open and feet at a stable distance. Having warned the patient, the medical examiner pulls on shoulders. In grade 0, a person is normal and not much affected. In grade one, a person stumbles but recovers on their own. By grade four, a person can no longer stand on their own.

Posture

A normal posture is erect. Grade one, the posture stoops. By grade four, Parkinson's causes extreme posture abnormality.

Rigidity

Seated, a person must perform a passive movement with the major joints. Grade one means slight motion difficulty. By grade four, rigidity is a severe problem.

Rapid alternating hand movements

In this test, a person must open and close as rapid as possible with alternating hands. In grade one, a person exhibits slow or slight amplitude reduction. By grade five, opening and closing their hands becomes an excruciating task.

Speech

Normal speech is grade 0, while a person experiences mild expression, diction, or volume issues by grade one. By grade four, a person becomes incoherent.

Tremor at rest

While the patient rests, the medical examiner grades the tremor in the head, upper, and lower extremities. Grade one shows occasional mild tremors. By grade four, a person suffers almost continuous tremors.

114

Trouble rising from a chair

Folding arms across chest, a patient must rise from a straight-back chair. In grade one, a person either stands slow or requires a second attempt. By grade four, they require help to get out of a chair.

UPDRS Part Four: Therapy Complications

A six question test, part four focuses on motor complications.

Part 4A: Dyskinesia

Before we review the test, let's turn to the Davis Phinney Foundation of Parkinson's disease to define Dyskinesia[141].

> *Dyskinesia literally means abnormal movement. Parkinson's Disease (PD) Dyskinesia, often referred to as levodopa-induced dyskinesia, can be described as uncontrolled jerking, dance-like, or wriggling movements. Symptoms range from minor tics to full-body movements. It can be a stand-alone condition; however, in people with Parkinson's, it is most often associated with long-term use of levodopa, a drug that increases levels of dopamine in the brain.*

Duration: What proportion of the waking day is dyskinesia present?

As in all tests, a 0 grade means normal, while grade 1 shows symptoms are present 1-25 percent of the day. The grades rise by 25 percent until dyskinesia is present 75-100 percent in grade four.

Disability: How disabling is the dyskinesia?

Doctors determine the level from historical information and by examination. A grade one means slight disability while one becomes 100% disabled by grade four.

Painful Dyskinesias: How painful is the dyskinesias?

Dyskinesia ranges from no pain in grade zero, to mild pain in grade one, to excruciating by grade four.

Early morning Dystonia

This question calls for a yes or no answer. A person either

experiences dystonia or not.

Part 4B: Clinical Fluctuations

What are clinical fluctuations?

> *A fluency disorder is an interruption in the flow of speaking characterized by an atypical rate, rhythm, and repetitions in sounds, syllables, words, and phrases.*
>
> *{Fluency disorders also cause} excessive tension, struggle behavior, and secondary mannerisms.*
>
> *–American Speech, Language, Hearing Association*[142]

Are off periods predictable?

Another yes or no answer.

Are off periods unpredictable?

Again, yes or no.

Are off periods sudden, within a few seconds?

Yes or no.

What proportion of the waking day is the patient off on average?

The grades range from zero to four, with zero meaning patient is normal, while one shows a 1-25% decline, and declines another 25% each grade until reaching 76-100% of the time in grade four.

Part 4C: Other Complications

Does the patient have anorexia, nausea, or vomiting?
Yes or no.

Any sleep disturbances, such as insomnia or hypersomnolence?
Yes or no.

Does the patient have symptomatic orthostasis?
Yes or no.

Additional Sources for Unified Parkinson's Disease Rating Scale (UPDRS): Wiley Online Library[143], Mayo Clinic[144], Kings College London[145], EPA[146], *Neurology*[147], *Academia*[148], University of Washington Medical Center[149]

Next, we will cover part five of the test, the Hoehn and Yahr Scale.

UPDRS Part Five: Hoehn and Yahr Scale

In 1968, Margaret Hoehn and Melvin Yahr developed the Hoehn and Yahr Scale and published in the Journal of Neurology[150].

Doctors still use the Hoehn and Yahr scale as one of two primary scales to determine Parkinson's stages.

As stated by the EPDA, the medical profession has since added three stages, stage 0, stage 1.5, and stage 2.5.

Early Stage

The early-stage covers stage one and part of stage two.

Stage 0

In stage 0, there are no Parkinson's symptoms.

Stage 1

Milder symptoms develop on one side of the body.

Stage 1.5

Unilateral symptoms, including the spine and neck.

Stage 2

Although no balance issues, in stage two, early symptoms show on both sides of the body.

Mid-Stage

Mid-stage indicates early-stage and mid-stage Parkinson's disease.

Stage 2.5

Symptoms advance on both sides, but a person can still pass a pull test, which is when a doctor stands behind and pulls the patient to test their balance. Even though other symptoms are advancing, a person can still balance during this stage.

Stage 3

In stage three, one's balance suffers, and other symptoms worsen. Parkinson's advances from mild to moderate.

Advanced-Stage

The disease becomes more debilitating in the advanced stage, including stages four and five.

Stage Four

By stage four, a person suffers significant mobility issues, but—with difficulty—a person can still stand and walk.

Stage Five

Stage five is the final act. A person becomes bedridden unless assisted in a wheelchair.

Parkinson's disease kills at the end of stage five, so there is no stage six. After stage five, we celebrate what I hope was a long, productive, and happy life.

***Hoehn and Yahr Scale Sources**: Parkinson's Resource Organization[151], Movement Disorder Society[152], U.S. Department of Veterans Affairs[153], Parkinson's Chronicles[154], and the Incidence and Prediction of falls in Parkinson's Disease study[155]*

Let's examine the Schwab and England Activities of Daily Living Scale.

UPDRS Part Six: Schwab and England Activities of Daily Living Scale

The Schwab and England Activities of Daily Living Scale measures Parkinson's decline in a sliding scale often. 100% is when no symptoms or difficulties show, whereas somebody reaches 0% when they reach a vegetable state, lose the ability to swallow, and organs quit.

100%

At 100%, a person exhibits no symptoms and remains independent and capable of performing normal daily duties. They remain oblivious there is a problem.

90%

At 90%, a person still can perform normal daily duties, but slower and with greater difficulty. A person notices something is wrong. Although not advanced, Parkinson's symptoms manifest and attack one's motor and non—motor skills. Whether they see the doctor (which they should!), they know of the symptoms.

80%

At 80%, a person remains independent and performs daily duties, although it takes twice as long and doubles the difficulty.

70%

Chores become more difficult to manage. No longer 100% independent. Struggles with chores, taking up to four times longer to complete. Chores that once took a few minutes will take an hour, and tasks once completed in an hour now take up an entire afternoon.

60%

At 60%, a Parkinson's disease patient struggles to perform chores, and cannot do some. Somebody must go behind them and refold clothes, wash dishes, dust, vacuum, etc.

50%

They continue to slow down in the chores they can do and require help with half what they once did themselves. Nothing comes easy anymore.

40%

Now dependent, the Parkinson's patient can no longer perform chores without help. At 40%, they require supervision to survive.

30%

At 30%, a dear one might attempt a chore, but the gaps grow longer, and their performance continues to slide. They require help or supervision to do anything.

20%

Dependent on others for everything. Might assist with a chore but is no longer capable of remembering how they once did things, nor can they learn tasks or grasp new concepts.

10%

At 10 percent, they lose whatever skills and abilities they maintained at 20%, and become invalid. They depend on others to eat, go to the bathroom, and almost every function, movement, and activity.

0%

At 0%, death is near. The organs shut down, and PDD patients cannot swallow. They are bedridden at this stage unless placed in a wheelchair and moved around.

Schwab and England Activities of Daily Living Scale Sources: BMC Neurology[156], U.S. Department of Veterans Affairs[157], Penn State University[158], A-Train Education[159]

Chapter 15:
CORTICOBASAL SYNDROME STAGES

To better understand symptoms, let's show how they manifest and develop from one stage to the next. This chapter divides corticobasal syndrome symptoms into three sections:

1. Early-stage
2. Mid-stage
3. Late-stage

I stress the symptoms and stages vary from one person to the next, but expect some variation of the following.

Early-stage Corticobasal Syndrome

The first sign might be something wrong involves an arm or hand in most cases. However, corticobasal syndrome apraxia also causes leg issues for some.

Damage to the frontal and temporal lobes breaks the neurological communication network between the brain and the arm, hand, or leg.

Depending on the severity level, one might experience stiffness, numbness, or near or total loss of feeling in the affected area.

Like a stroke victim, some with corticobasal syndrome gives the brain command to move a hand, arm, or leg, but the signal does not fire like a short in an electrical wire, the damaged neurons, and synapses.

Synapses work somewhat like the internet, creating a chemical signal allowing neurons to communicate and share information throughout the body

Below are possible early CBS symptoms, although some of these happen in the mid-stage for many.

Early-state Symptoms List

- Acalculia
- Akinesia
- Alien limb phenomenon
- Apraxia
- Bradykinesia
- Dystonia
- Visuospatial disorder

Early-stage corticobasal syndrome symptoms focus primarily on an arm or hand, and with less frequency in a leg.

Mid-stage Corticobasal Syndrome

In mid-stage, early-stage symptoms worsen, and new symptoms develop.

Mid-stage symptoms list

- Acalculia (cannot compute basic math)
- Aphasia (speech and language deterioration)
- Impaired executive skills (struggles to plan or carry out basic tasks)
- Memory loss (short-term)
- Unable to adapt to the unexpected
- Visuospatial disorder (No longer able to process the world. Cannot locate objects surrounding them)

For those who struggled with basic math in stage one, doing so at some point in stage two becomes impossible. Stage one bradykinesia problems cause even slower movement in stage two.

The alien limb phenomenon worsens in stage two, causing immeasurable anxiety. Think of how doctors use a rubber mallet to tap your knee and produce the knee-jerk (patellar reflex). Parts of your body move similarly, but without any prompt from a doctor's mallet or your brain's command. Uncontrolled movements grow worse. This symptom alone produces a wide variety of emotional stress.

On the opposite spectrum, apraxia problems also grow more severe. Think of things people learn as a child and develop the rest of our lives, such as moving our arms or hands. As the damage to the brain grows worse, the symptoms grow more severe, including one's inability to perform learned motor skills.

Dystonia (uncontrolled muscle contractions) exacerbate in stage two. Those who suffer Alien limb phenomenon, aphaxia, and dystonia already delivered a triple dose of agony, discomfort, and disability. But the trio threat only represents a portion of their suffering.

The visuospatial system deteriorates more in stage two, destroying one's place in the world and rendering them helpless to recognize objects in their general vicinity.

By stage two, corticobasal syndrome patients cannot adapt to the unexpected. Too many symptoms overwhelm them at once, so it takes all one can manage to address the normal and expected.

Stage two destroys any remaining executive skills.

While most Corticobasal syndrome patients avoid short-term memory loss in stage one, such cognitive issues become more prominent in stage two.

Unfortunately, stage two is only a prelude for stage three. Science does not yet offer a model where the stages show improvement, but instead a slow, unsteady march towards the end.

Late-stage Corticobasal Syndrome

Disoriented. Pumped full of anxiety. Depressed. Overwhelmed. One arrives at late-stage corticobasal syndrome suffering a great many physical symptoms and a variety of emotional pain.

Stage one and two symptoms provided immeasurable challenges for the corticobasal syndrome patient and loved ones. By this point, one needs help getting in and out of bed or going to the bathroom. Many require a wheelchair by this stage.

Rapid and constant blinking is characteristic of late-stage corticobasal syndrome.

Communicating grows increasingly difficult, as language skills deterioration continues.

By late stage, dementia grows more prominent, shattering short-term memory, destroying remaining executive skills, and sending people into a cognitive nosedive.

Corticobasal Syndrome (CBS) Cause of Death

As with most dementias, corticobasal syndrome (CBS) does not directly kill most people. Instead, CBS produces a smorgasbord of progressive symptoms, weakening the body and destroying the mind.

Swallowing issues cause many problems, some life-threatening such as pneumonia and chest infections from swallowing food particles down the wrong pipe into the lungs.

According to the Association for Frontotemporal Degeneration, "Death in CBS is generally caused by pneumonia or other complications, such as sepsis (infection throughout the body) or pulmonary embolism (a blood clot that blocks a major blood vessel in the lung)[160]."

The average corticobasal syndrome patient lives six to eight years from the time symptoms manifest.

Additional Symptoms & Stages Sources: National Health Service[161], Association for Frontotemporal Degeneration[162], Annals of Research Hospitals[163]

IV. LEWY BODY DEMENTIA/PARKINSONISM RISK FACTORS

This chapter covers risk factors for dementia with Lewy bodies (DLB), Parkinson's disease dementia (PDD), and corticobasal syndrome.

As with symptoms, the three dementias share some but not all risk factors.

Chapter 16: DLB RISK FACTORS

As with most dementia, we do not know the cause of the Lewy body dementias. Studies, however, point to risk factors we cover in this chapter.

We list the risk factors, then discuss them one by one. When we view the risk factors for most major noncommunicable diseases, we see the usual suspects.

What are the risk factors for Dementia with Lewy Bodies?

1. Age[164]
2. Anxiety[165]
3. Cancer history[166]
4. Chemical exposure[167]
5. Depression[168]
6. Gender[169]
7. Heredity[170]
8. High blood sugar & high blood pressure[171]
9. Low caffeine consumption[172]
10. Mental Inactivity[173]
11. Parkinson's disease
12. Physical inactivity[42]
13. Pesticides exposure[174]
14. Sleep disorders[175]
15. Strokes[176]
16. Tobacco[177]
17. Unhealthy diet[178]
18. Vitamin deficiency[179]

We can eliminate most of the causes through better habits. The more we investigate dementia and modern diseases, the more apparent the average human is on a slow, or not so slow suicidal march. But, we hold control over most causes.

Let's see how this list compares to Parkinson's disease dementia risk factors.

Parkinson's Disease Dementia (PDD) Risk Factors

1. Age
2. Anxiety
3. Chemical exposure
4. Depression
5. Ethnicity
6. Gender
7. Family history/genetics[180]
8. Formal education
9. Head trauma
10. Hypertension & high blood pressure
11. Low caffeine consumption
12. Mental Inactivity
13. Obesity
14. Physical inactivity
15. Pesticides and herbicide exposure
16. Sleep disorders
17. Strokes
18. Unhealthy diet
19. Vitamin deficiency

When reviewing the list, the first thing that jumps out is we indeed hold some control over most of these risk factors. The second is the risk factors are similar to dementia with Lewy bodies (DLB).

Corticobasal Syndrome (CBS) Risk Factors

UCSF Weill Institute for Neurosciences describes corticobasal syndrome's (CBS) underlying pathology.

> *The cause of CBS is unknown. Scientists know that in some people with CBS, there is a large build-up of a protein called **tau**. Tau occurs normally in the brain, but we do not yet understand what causes it to build up in large amounts. Others may have a large build-up of amyloid plaques similar to those seen in people with Alzheimer's disease. As more and more proteins build up in the nerve cells, the cells lose their ability to function and eventually die. This causes affected parts of the brain to shrink[181].*

As UCSF points out, CBS cause remains unknown. While I wish this were uncommon, the cause remains mysterious for several dementias.

In most dementias, science understands what happens, but not why. Protein deposits or tangles are front and center of the neuron damage resulting in CBS, Alzheimer's, and other dementias. But, many neurologists argue the protein buildup is a defense response, not the cause.

Science confirms most CBS is sporadic, meaning you do not inherit the disorder from a parent. However, other than pointing towards tau and amyloid protein, humans remain in the dark concerning CBS cause and risk factors.

We will update the corticobasal syndrome risk factors once science unveils others. For now, corticobasal shares age as a risk factor with Parkinson's disease dementia (PDD) and dementia with Lewy bodies (DLB).

133

Age

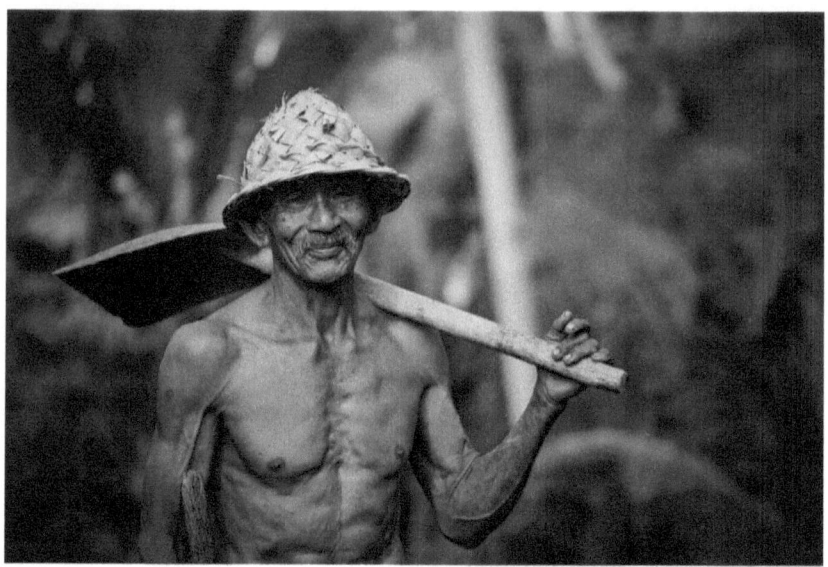

Although the disease can strike earlier, advanced age is the "greatest risk factor for Lewy body dementia, with onset typically, but not always, between the ages of 50 and 85," according to the Lewy Body Dementia Association[182].

Parkinson's disease manifests in most people in their sixties, although 15% of Parkinson's cases are under forty[183]. Parkinson's disease dementia develops in the average Parkinson's patient age 65 or older.

As we age, the risks increase for dementia and other fatal diseases.

However, we hold a great influence on how we age. I'm not talking about dying hair, getting nose jobs, or other cosmetic attempts to look younger or prettier, but life choices that slow the aging process. To some extent, we are the result of our habits, so establish healthy ones.

The recipe for graceful aging is the same for everybody. Avoid or minimize stress, depression & anxiety. Eat a balanced whole food diet and get 7-8 hours' sleep per night.

Enjoy the sunrises, sunsets, rainbows, moon, stars, and nature. Exercise 4-7 days per week and make it fun. Practice the Golden Rule. We encounter fewer problems when we treat others right.

Anxiety

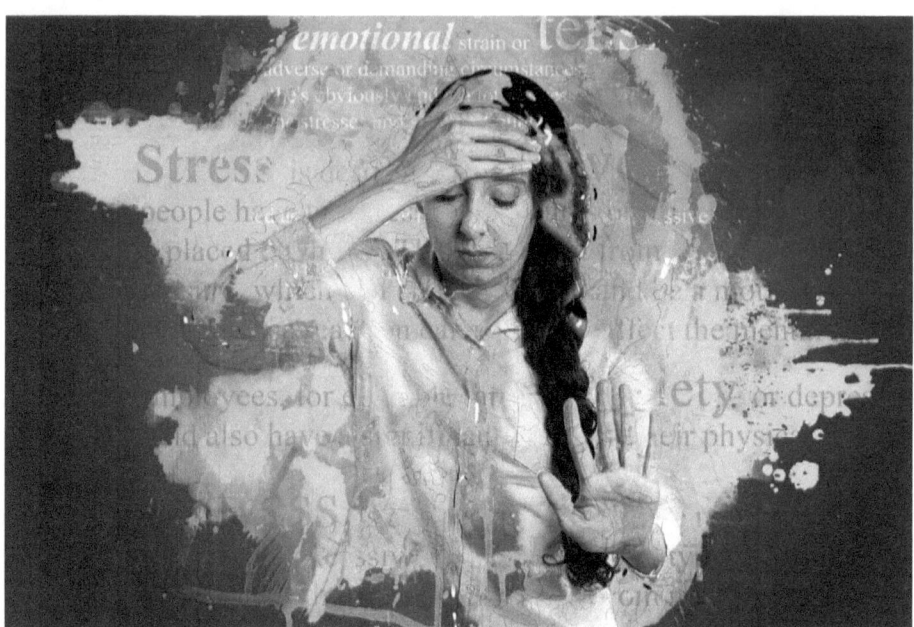

We know anxiety plays a role in both forms of Lewy body dementia, but need more studies to determine whether anxiety is a risk factor or symptom.

Anxiety shows early in most Lewy body dementia cases, which complicates uncovering its association with the disease. A study released in *PubMed* analyzed risk factors for dementia with Lewy bodies. "Compared with controls, subjects with DLB were more likely to have a history of anxiety[184]," the study concluded.

Other studies confirm a relationship between anxiety and both Lewy body dementias but have yet to confirm which is the risk factor or symptom.

A study of 174,776 people released in *PubMed* found anxiety disorders increase Parkinson's disease risks[185]. They concluded the greater the anxiety, the greater the risk.

Director of Johns Hopkins Parkinson's Disease

Neuropsychiatry Clinic, Gregory Pontone, M.D. addressed anxiety's link to PD. "It may be that anxiety disorders that are diagnosed as much as two decades before Parkinson's disease may be a harbinger of the disease," said Pontone.

> *One theory is that the anxiety that comes before Parkinson's results from the same underlying changes in brain chemistry and circuitry. Others believe that Parkinson's disease and anxiety share a common genetic risk factor. Either way, taking a closer look at the link can help doctors understand the causes of Parkinson's and treat patients with the disease[186].*

The Parkinson's Outcomes Project[187] conducted the largest clinical study of Parkinson's disease covering five countries. They concluded anxiety and depression "play a key role in the disease as well and its effect on people's quality of life[188]."

Studies link anxiety as a risk factor and symptom, not uncommon for neurological disorders. We need more studies to confirm the exact relationship, but anxiety plays a large role in PDD.

Chemical exposure

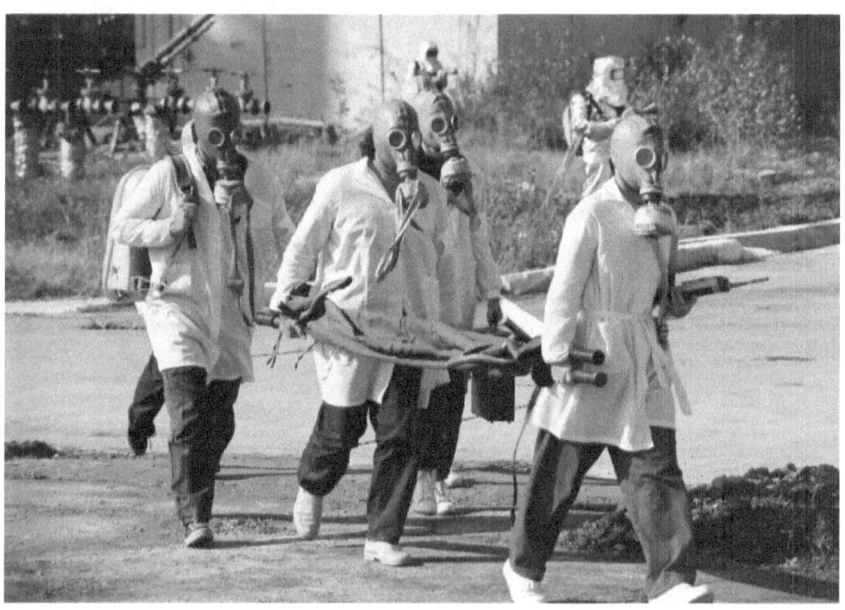

Some scientists and studies point to chemical exposure as a risk factor for Parkinson's disease and Lewy body dementia.

One study released in PubMed investigated the link between toxins in the environment and Parkinson's disease.

Overall, all this body of evidence strongly suggests that environmental toxins may play an important role in the appearance and progression of PD pathology. This is especially true for iPD. In these patients, the progression of the pathology may start from the ENS and OB and follows a predictable spatiotemporal pattern. Interestingly, these are the two nervous structures most exposed to environmental toxins and in vitro and in vivo studies suggest that environmental toxins acting on the ENS could initiate the pathology and trigger its progression through the release and transcellular transport of alpha-synuclein[52].

A review by Samuel M. Goldman, M.D. from the Parkinson's Institute concluded: "Epidemiologic studies have found an increased risk of PD associated with exposure to environmental toxicants such as pesticides, solvents, metals, and other pollutants, and many of these compounds recapitulate PD pathology in animal models[189]."

While we need more studies, chemical exposure plays a role in the development of Parkinson's, Alzheimer's, dementia with Lewy bodies, and other dementias. We need large controlled human studies to determine how large a role chemical toxins play as a dementia risk factor.

While waiting for more studies to confirm which toxins increase the risk, it is best to watch the chemicals we expose ourselves to around our house.

We might have limited or no control over toxins in our workplace and other public places, but we can remove toxins from our homes. Natural products exist, and some work as well or better than their toxin-filled counterparts.

Depression

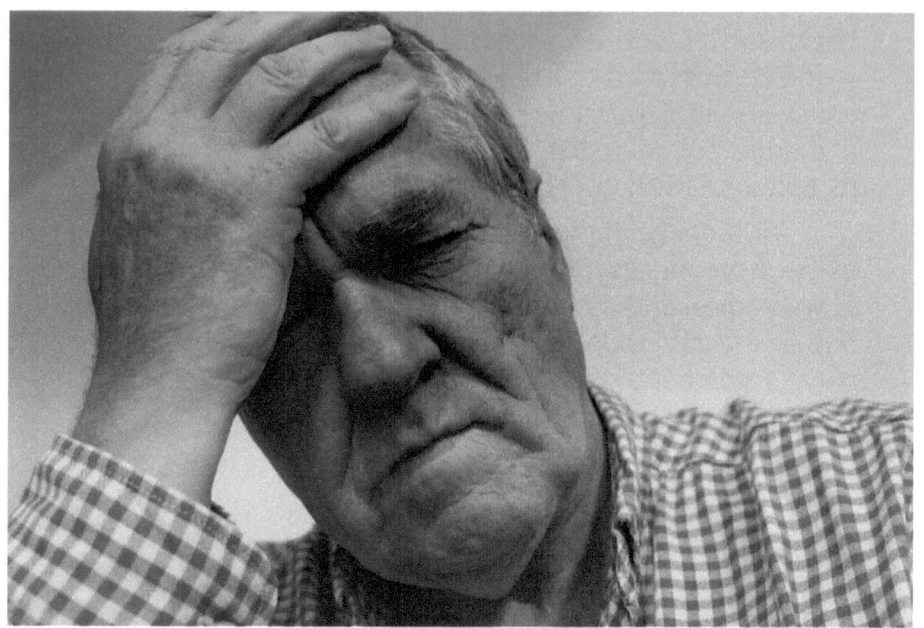

Depression, like anxiety, connects to dementia with Lewy bodies, but is it a risk factor or symptom?

"Anxiety and depression may be early indicators of disease onset, or they may also be a natural response to mild cognitive decline," the LBDA reported. "Yet, in people who do not have symptoms during life, but have Lewy body pathology in their brains at autopsy, anxiety and depression are uncommon[190]."

I scratched my head after reading the paragraph, and reread, hoping I had misread the LBDA report.

"Perhaps these symptoms increase the likelihood that someone seeks a doctor for an evaluation," the LBDA added. "Further research is needed to identify features that may aid in a pre-dementia diagnosis of DLB."

A respective cohort study followed subgroups of people diagnosed with depression from 1975 to 1990, and then in 2000 conducted a follow-up. The researchers published their results in *Neurology* in 2002, finding "A strong positive association between depression and subsequent incidence of Parkinson's disease[191]."

A more recent nationwide cohort study followed 140,688 people suffering from depression. The study's lead author Helena Gustafsson, MD., Department of Community Medicine and Rehabilitation, Geriatrics noted Parkinson's patients suffer greater levels of depression than people without PD.

Like Alzheimer's, Parkinson's develops for a long period before symptoms manifest. Does depression play a role?

"Given that the association was significant for a follow-up period of more than two decades," said Gustafsson, "depression may be a very early prodromal symptom of PD or a causal risk factor[192]."

We will not develop cures for Alzheimer's and Parkinson's disease until a better understanding of what takes place before the symptoms leading to diagnosis. Nor will there likely be one cure for Parkinson's because we must address all risk factors, which requires a combination of lifestyle changes, vaccines, and other means of addressing the underlining factors causing PDD.

The connection between depression and PD is strong and requires more research. Defeating PD requires addressing these many underlying causes, such as anxiety and depression before they do permanent damage.

Anxiety and depression may or may not increase one's risk for dementia with Lewy bodies or Parkinson's disease dementia, but there are almost as many reasons to avoid or minimize both as there is to quit smoking. If they do not kill you one way, they will find another.

Ethnicity

A 2009 Department of Neurology, University of Pennsylvania study published in PubMed found whites are far more likely to get Parkinson's disease than African-Americans and Latinos. The study concluded the following PD percentages[193]:

67%   White

28%   African American

4%   Latino

Why such a gap?

Parkinson's disease may be"under-recognized in African-Americans based on this data, but it remains uncertain why," said lead author Nabila Dahodwala, M.D.

What about Latinos? The Latino number stands out even more than 28% for African Americans.

One explanation might be higher mortality rates for African-Americans and Latinos due to diabetes and other diseases.

Let's view the *Geographic and Ethnic Variation in Parkinson's Disease* study. Comparing Parkinson's rates per 100,000, the researchers concluded:

16.17 White

11.38   Asian

10.36 African-American

What's the study's importance?

"Parkinson disease is substantially more common in whites,' said lead author Allison Wright Willis, "and is nonrandomly distributed in the Midwest and Northeastern US.

Not certain why the researchers did not include Asians in the first study, or the authors grouped Hispanics either with whites or African-Americans.

The studies thus far suggest PD attacks whites in far greater numbers than other ethnicities.

Let's dig deeper.

A Division of Research, Kaiser Permanente study also measured ethnic Parkinson's incidence per 100,000 people. They found[194]:

16.6   Hispanics

13.6   Whites

11.3   Asians

10.2   African-Americans

The results show similar numbers for whites, Asians, and blacks from the *Geographic and Ethnic Variation in Parkinson's Disease* study, but much higher numbers for Hispanics than the first study cited.

Researchers must figure out why, but—from the information available—Hispanics and non-Hispanic whites suffer much higher rates of Parkinson's disease than Asians or African-Americans.

Family History

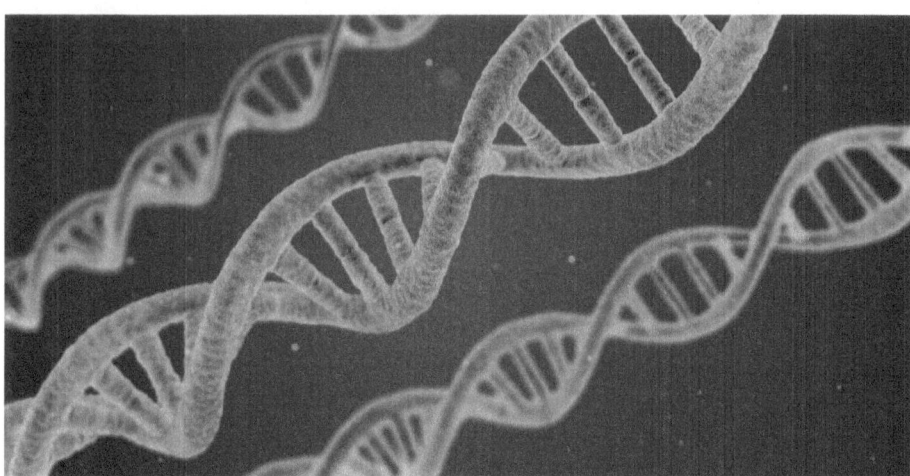

If a family member has either version, one is more likely to get Dementia with Lewy bodies and Parkinson's disease dementia.

According to the National Institute of Neurological Disorders and Strokes (NIH), "having a family member with LBD may increase a person's risk, LBD is not normally considered a genetic disease."

How many families carry this risk?

"A small percentage of families with dementia with Lewy bodies has a genetic association, such as a variant of the GBA gene," said NIH, "but in most cases, the cause is unknown[195]."

While the families who carry the GBA gene variant carry a higher risk, this affects only a small percentage of families.

If you have a family member with Lewy body dementia, take the same steps, everybody else should minimize this substantial risk factor.

Genetics

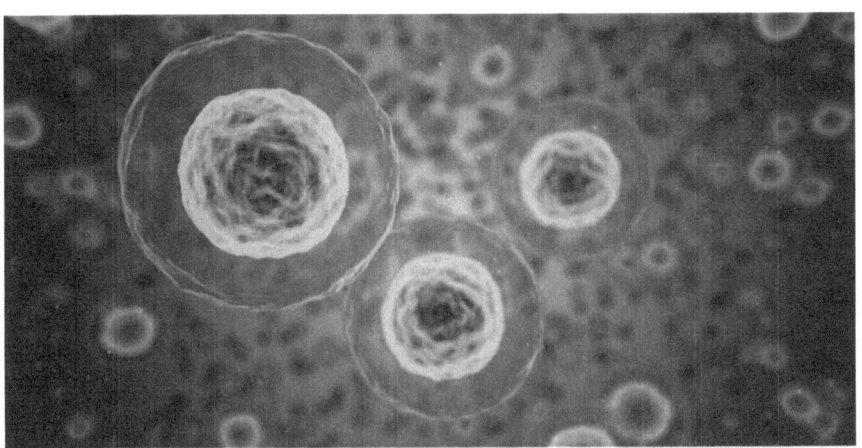

Genetics causes about 10% of Lewy body dementia cases[196].

SNCA and SNCB gene mutations

SNCA and SNCB provide the system a recipe for making the alpha-synuclein and beta-synuclein proteins.

The **SNCA** *and* **SNCB** *genes provide instructions for making proteins, called alpha-synuclein and beta-synuclein, respectively, that are found primarily in the brain. Alpha-synuclein plays a role in communication between nerve cells (neurons), helping to regulate the release of chemical messengers* (neurotransmitters). *Beta-synuclein is likely involved in a process that allows neurons to change and adapt over time, which is necessary for learning and memory. Beta-synuclein may also prevent {a} harmful accumulation of alpha-synuclein in neurons[63].*

−U.S. National Library of Medicine[197]

SNCA (Synuclein Alpha)

The Human Gene Database associates SNCA with Parkinson's disease and dementia with Lewy bodies. "Among its related pathways are Parkinson's Disease Pathway and Respiratory electron transport, ATP synthesis by chemiosmotic coupling, and heat production by uncoupling proteins[198]."

What about SNCB?

SNCB (Synuclein Beta)

A protein-coding gene, SNCB[199] (Synuclein Beta), is associated with Parkinson's disease dementia and dementia with Lewy bodies. The gene's responsibilities include binding alpha-tubulin and calcium ion.

While not present in Lewy bodies, scientists believe Beta-synuclein is an alpha-synuclein connected to Parkinson's disease, dementia with Lewy bodies, and other neurodegenerative diseases[200]. The working theory is beta-synuclein protects the central nervous system from alpha-synuclein neurotoxins[201].

Formal education

Whereas lower formal education increases odds for Alzheimer's, some studies suggest the opposite effect on Parkinson's disease.

A study in Sweden released on *PubMed* compared four decades of data and found a low level of formal education reduces one's risk of Parkinson's disease[202].

Another *PubMed* study drew opposite conclusions, but suggested IQ might play a larger role than education[203].

A Mayo Clinic study published in the *American Academy of Neurology*[204] found a higher risk factor for Parkinson's disease in those with nine or more years of education, and higher the education level, the higher the risk.

Why do the studies draw conflicting results?

The most probable answer is the studies do not account for

other factors. Perhaps, IQ is more important as the *PubMed* study suggests.

Mayo Clinic study lead-author Roberta Frigerio, MD, weighed in on the debate. "These factors may be surrogates for a variety of exposures, physical activity, personality, or socioeconomic status," said Frigerio. "Further studies are needed to interpret our findings[205]."

Another reason for the contrasting studies is not all people in either group are the same. If a person with high formal education eats a poor diet, exercises little or none, allows stress to evolve into anxiety, does not get enough sleep, and otherwise develops unhealthy habits, their high formal education will not save them.

Similar, if a person with a low level of formal education eats a healthy diet, exercises, avoid stress, read books, socialize, and otherwise practices healthy habits, they reduce their odds of Parkinson's and other diseases.

That so many in our culture have low formal education or stop learning indicts individuals and society.

However, that lower educated people reduce their risks of Parkinson's and other diseases through healthy habits confirm them for everybody.

Gender

Men and women are best together, but we are different.

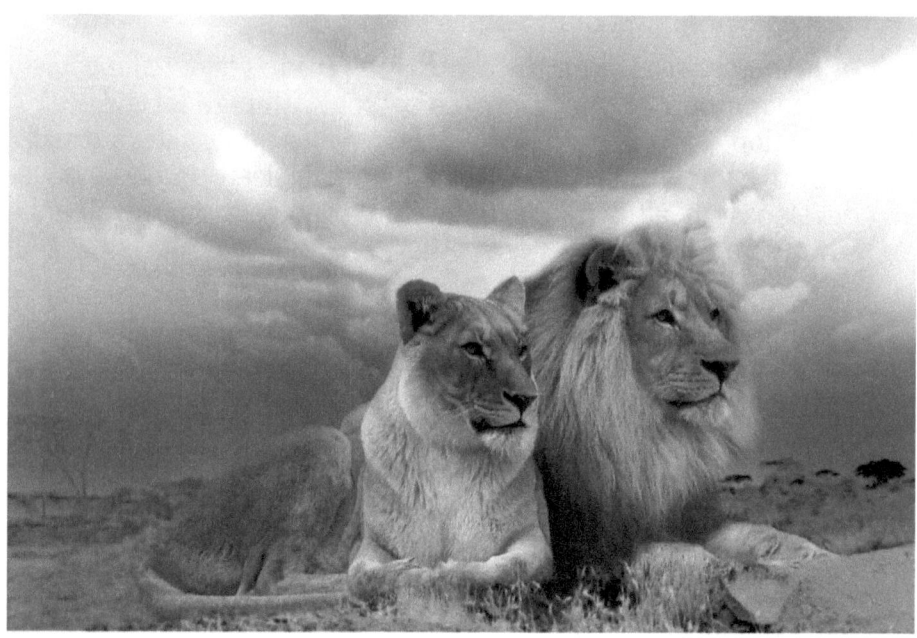

Men are more likely to get Lewy body dementia than women. A study released in Pub Med reviewed dozens of studies measuring gender's role in Lewy body dementia.

Lead author, Peter T. Nelson, Division of Neuropathology, Department of Pathology, Sanders-Brown Center on Aging, University of Kentucky, explained the study's findings.

"Data from large autopsy series indicate that there is a positive association between male gender and risk for dying with relatively 'pure' cortical DLB pathology," said Nelson. "This effect does not appear to be related to potential confounders such as patients' age of death, education level, smoking status, or ApoE alleles[206]."

How did the studies stack against other research?

"Prior American, European, and Japanese autopsy series," said Nelson, "have found disproportionate numbers of males in pathologically confirmed DLB cohorts."

An autopsy study by the University of Pennsylvania concluded men are almost three times more likely than women to get Lewy body dementia[207].

Other studies suggest men are 1.5 to 3 times likelier than women to get Lewy body dementia. While we need deeper studies to determine the exact percentage, men are more likely to get dementia with Lewy bodies, Parkinson's disease, and Parkinson's disease dementia than women.

Head Trauma

The possible connection between head trauma and Parkinson's is illustrated — perhaps nowhere more prominently — by Muhammad Ali's diagnosis of young-onset Parkinson's disease (PD) following a career in boxing. Many have wondered whether repeated hits to the head caused his PD. While it's true that environmental factors — including head injury — have been associated with an increased risk of Parkinson's, few (if any) have been determined to be definitive causes of the disease. Environmental factors and genetics may interact to cause disease, and this complex interplay makes it virtually impossible to point to the exact cause(s) in any individual.

Michael J. Fox Foundation for Parkinson's Research

A group of Faculty of Medicine, University of British Columbia Neurologists, reviewed 636 articles and narrowed it down to meet three standards. One, the studies must include confirmed PD patients. Two, the studies must include verified head trauma, causing concussions. Three, the studies must include odds ratios or 95% or greater confidence intervals. The research team released its review on PubMed.

The team concluded: "Our meta-analysis indicates that a history of head trauma that results in concussion is associated with a higher risk of developing PD[208]."

The Parkinson's Institute conducted a controlled case study, including 93 twin pairs. "Our results suggest that mild-to-moderate closed head injury may increase PD risk decades later," said Samuel Goldman, MD, MPH, UCSF School of

Medicine[209].

Another study released in the Annals of Neurology concluded traumatic brain injury "is associated with a 44% increased risk of developing PD over 5 to 7 years that is unlikely to be due to confounding or reverse causation[210]."

The three cited and several other studies confirm traumatic brain injuries elevate PDD risk, but as the Michael J. Fox Foundation emphasized, somebody prone to Parkinson's might suffer greater trauma and head injuries than others.

Hypertension & High Blood Pressure

High blood pressure increases the risk of heart attack, chronic heart failure, kidney disease, and strokes. According to the CDC, high blood pressure is the primary or contributing cause of daily deaths for 1,000 Americans[211].

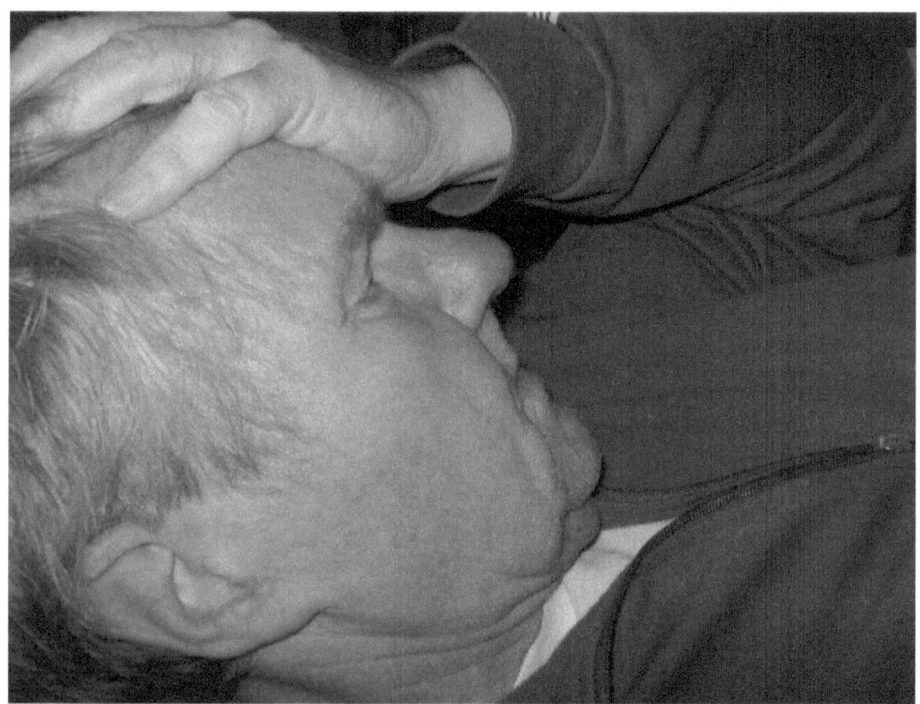

Do you or a health professional monitor your blood pressure?

The CDC claims high blood pressure increases the risk of Parkinson's disease and dementia.

A University of Michigan cohort study of 275 Parkinson's patients with early symptoms found elevated systolic blood pressure increase the risk of motor disability and severity in Parkinson's patients[212].

While this does not prove high blood pressure, lead author

Christina Lineback exuberated in her presentation to the 68th annual meeting of the American Academy of Neurology.

"Identifying clinical features associated with more aggressive disease progression in Parkinson's disease, such as blood pressure, may be important in future studies," said Lineback. "Researchers may begin to incorporate these baseline prognostic markers into the randomization stage of future clinical trials."

A meta-analysis of 27 observational studies, including 1,230,085 participants in North America, Europe, or Asia, concluded: "Based on population-based cohort studies, this meta-analysis indicated that hypertension might increase the risk of PD[213]."

While most studies show high blood pressure increases Parkinson's risk, a minority did not find any significant difference. What we know for certain is high blood pressure worsens motor problems associated with Parkinson's disease.

Like diabetes, high blood pressure is systematic of modern life and elevates risks for heart disease, cancer, dementia, and many other life-threatening disorders

Almost half of Americans have high blood pressure because of poor diets, lack of exercise, and corresponding weight issues.

How is blood pressure measured?

We gauge blood pressure by measuring two pressures, systolic (top number) and diastolic (bottom number).

Systolic Pressure

Systolic pressure measures artery and blood vessels pressure per heartbeat.

Diastolic Pressure

Diastolic pressure measures the pressure between heartbeats.

What is normal blood pressure, high blood pressure, and hypertension?

New Blood Pressure Reading Measurements

The American Heart Association established new guidelines for blood pressure readings. Let's review the chart of their updated recommendations:

BP Category	Systolic BP mm Hg (upper number)		Diastolic BP mm hg (lower number)
Normal	Under 120	&	Under 80
Elevated	120-129	&	Under 80
Hypertension: Stage 1	130-139	or	80-89
Hypertension: Stage 2	140 or over	or	90 or over
Hypertension: Emergency	Over 180	&/or	Over 120

Source: *American College of Cardiology/American Heart Association Task Force on Clinical Practice Guidelines[214].*

The new guidelines lower maximum levels allowed for normal, elevated, and hypertension blood pressure.

There are many reasons to manage your blood pressure, but lowering your dementia risks ranks high. If high blood pressure does not increase risks for Parkinson's disease dementia, and dementia with Lewy bodies, the strokes and heart disease it causes do.

Next, let's view a risk that might surprise most people.

Low Caffeine Consumption

Authorities have warned us for decades to minimize our caffeine consumption.

Several studies suggest higher caffeine use might provide health benefits. However, other studies suggest the opposite[215]. What gives?

The way we consume caffeine varies. Studies of coffee[216] [217] and tea[218] consumption bring positive results[219], while synthetic caffeine in a pill or other drinks shows less impressive outcomes.

With that distinction, some studies suggest coffee and tea consumption might lower risks for Parkinson's disease and dementia with Lewy bodies.

The advice does not suggest you should drink coffee until your eyes bulge and shake from head to toe. Nor should you think oversized soft drinks are the answer.

From the evidence available, drink and enjoy coffee and tea if it causes no other health issues[220]. Coffee is best black and unsweetened (enjoy the bold, uncorrupted flavor), and the tea unsweetened.

A genetic study suggests drinking coffee might provide your offspring and descendants protection against Parkinson's and other diseases. The study, released in *Molecular Psychiatry*, found "the role of caffeine in mediating habitual coffee consumption and may point to molecular mechanisms underlying inter-individual variability in pharmacological and health effects of coffee[221]."

One last note.

The information here is for reducing the risks of getting Parkinson's or dementia, and might not produce the same benefits once somebody has Parkinson's disease[222].

For those who do not have Parkinson's or dementia, enjoy a cup of coffee or tea. Green tea is a great option, but both boost health benefits.

Pesticides Exposure

We dump tons of chemicals per year to keep insects from eating crops or sharing our homes, shops, and workplaces. Deep down, we know some of these chemicals are dangerous, but our societal insect phobia drives us to suicidal tendencies.

The insecticides, herbicides, fungicides, and other chemicals end up in our water, food, air, clothing, homes, workplaces, and almost everywhere we visit.

Do these chemicals increase our risk for Parkinson's disease and dementia with Lewy bodies?

Paraquat and Rotenone

A study published in *Environmental Health Perspectives* conducted a lifetime assessment of paraquat and rotenone. They concluded Parkinson's disease is: "positively associated with two groups of pesticides defined by mechanisms implicated experimentally—those that impair mitochondrial function and those that increase oxidative stress, supporting a role for these mechanisms in PD pathophysiology[223]."

Paraquat

The "highly poisonous" paraquat is a category one herbicide toxin[224].

In the seventies and eighties, the United States government weaponized paraquat in their misguided war against marijuana. The American government sprayed marijuana plants with paraquat in Mexico, Columbia, and other countries south of the border[225]. They also used it in Georgia[226] in the United States. Even the maker of the company objected to the use of his product in such a manner.

Recognizing the dangers, the United States banned the use of paraquat for all but commercial use by licensed applicators.

Studies confirm paraquat produces oxidative stress, reactive oxygen species (ROS), and an aggregate of a-synucleins[227] in neurons[228].

A study released in Nature Chemical Biology identified the

three genes attacked by paraquat leading to Parkinson's disease:

- *POR* (cytochrome P450 oxidoreductase)
- *ATP7A* (copper transporter)
- *SLC45A4* (sucrose transporter)

The researchers determined paraquat attacks all three genes through oxidative stress causing dopamine neuron damage.

Rotenone

Colorless and odorless, rotenone is a natural insecticide and pesticide used in many households. Researchers consider controlled dosages safe, but warn rotenone turns toxic in high doses[229].

A *Journal of Neuroscience* study created a rotenone model of PD and added to the evidence connecting rotenone to Parkinson's disease. They concluded: "(1) that rotenone acts specifically at complex I, and (2) that oxidative damage, strongly implicated in PD pathogenesis, plays a pivotal role in rotenone toxicity both in vivo and in vitro[230]."

NIEHS researcher and lead author of another study, Freya Kamel, Ph.D., explained rotenone's relationship to Parkinson's disease.

"Rotenone directly inhibits the function of the mitochondria, the structure responsible for making energy in the cell," said Kamel. "Paraquat increases the production of certain oxygen derivatives that may harm cellular structures. People who used these pesticides or others with a similar mechanism of action were more likely to develop Parkinson's disease[231]."

While researchers linked paraquat and rotenone to Parkinson's disease, they call for more studies to identify other pesticides and chemicals, increasing PD risk.

Let's now view how sleep disorders increase one's risk of dementia with Lewy bodies.

Sleep disorder

We require 7-8 hours of sleep per night for optimum health. Parkinson's disease patients might find no difficulty falling to sleep but wake within a couple of hours, unable to fall back to sleep. They often awake to go to the bathroom, suffer restless leg syndrome, find it difficult to roll over, and experience nightmares and vivid dreams[232]. They feel tired during the day and suffer maintenance insomnia.

Researchers connect this to Hcrt cells.

What is Hcrt?

"This gene encodes a hypothalamic neuropeptide precursor protein that gives rise to two mature neuropeptides, orexin A and orexin B, by proteolytic processing," said NCBI. "Orexin A and orexin B, which bind to orphan G-protein-coupled receptors HCRTR1 and HCRTR2, function {regulating} sleep and arousal[233]."

How are Hcrt cells related to Parkinson's disease or dementia with Lewy bodies?

UCLA/Veteran Affairs Study

A team of UCLA and Veteran Affairs, Parkinson's disease researchers, discovered a connection between narcolepsy and Parkinson's. Narcolepsy is a disorder caused by damaged orexin/hypocretin (Hcrt) cells[234].

Study author Jerry Siegel, Ph.D., professor of psychiatry and biobehavioral sciences at the Semel Institute for Neuroscience and Human Behavior at UCLA, reported the findings.

"We found that PD is characterized by a massive loss of Hcrt neurons," said Siegel. "Thus, {losing} Hcrt cells may be a cause of the narcolepsy-like symptoms of PD and may be {improved} by treatments aimed at reversing the Hcrt deficit."

Siegel claims Parkinson's patients lose 60% of the peptide hypocretin brain cells.

What else did the study uncover?

"We also saw a substantial loss of hypothalamic MCH neurons," said Doctor Siegel. "The losses of Hcrt and MCH neurons are significantly correlated with the clinical stage of PD, not disease duration, whereas {losing} neuromelanin cells is significantly correlated only with disease duration."

Why is this important?

"The significant correlations we found between the loss of Hcrt and MCH neurons and the clinical stage of PD," said Siegel, "in contrast to the lack of a relationship of similar strength between a loss of neuromelanin containing cells and the clinical symptoms of PD, suggests a previously unappreciated relationship between hypothalamic dysfunction and the time course of the overall clinical picture of PD."

Parkinson's disease produces many types of disorders. Many experts point to RBD as the greatest concern.

RBD

REM (Restless Eye Movement) Sleep behavior Disorder (RBD) disrupts the paralysis separating us from our dreams, causing us to react to our dreams. They are engaged in their dreams and, in their minds, defending themselves from attackers, monsters, or whatever their dream world produces. People scream, cuss, threaten, shriek, snarl, swing, kick, attack, run and otherwise respond to whoever or whatever threatens them in a deep mysterious part of their mind.

According to the Mayo Clinic, RBD (REM sleep behavior disorder) relates to both Parkinson's disease and dementia with Lewy bodies[235].

Almost 60% of those with Parkinson's disease and 80-100% of dementia with Lewy bodies patients have RBD[236].

Systematic Review of PDD Risk Factors Studies

A review posted in BMC[237] screened 5,195 studies and found 25 matching their criteria to determine risk factors for Parkinson's disease dementia.

The researchers concluded, "Advanced age, male, higher

UPDRS III scores, hallucination, RBD, smoking, and hypertension increase the risk of PDD, whereas higher education is a protective factor for PDD[238]."

Denmark Study

Researchers in Denmark study concluded people suffering RBD disorders: "have an inflammation of the brain in the area {around} the dopamine-producing nerve cells[239]."

The discovery pertains directly to people experiencing RBD risk Parkinson's disease or dementia with Lewy bodies.

"They already suffer from a lack of dopamine in the brain," the researchers explained in a press release. "Parkinson's disease occurs precisely because the group of nerve cells in the brain that produce dopamine stop working[240]."

Make sleeping 7.5-8.5 hours a priority. If you suffer any sleep disorder, see a doctor, but try to solve the problem without medication. You should avoid sleep drugs, including over-the-counter, unless a last resort. The lesson in disease after disease, study after study is how crucial it is to get a good night's sleep.

We will next analyze stroke's connection to Parkinson's disease and dementia with Lewy bodies.

Strokes

Strokes cause 2-5.5% of Parkinson's disease, and the name is Vascular Parkinsonism[241].

According to Baylor College of Medicine[242]:

Vascular (also referred to as "multi-infarct") parkinsonism is a form of "atypical parkinsonism" in which parkinsonian symptoms (slow movements, tremor, difficulty with walking and balance, stiffness and rigidity) are produced by one or more small strokes, rather than by gradual loss of nerve cells as seen in the more typical neurodegenerative Parkinson's disease.

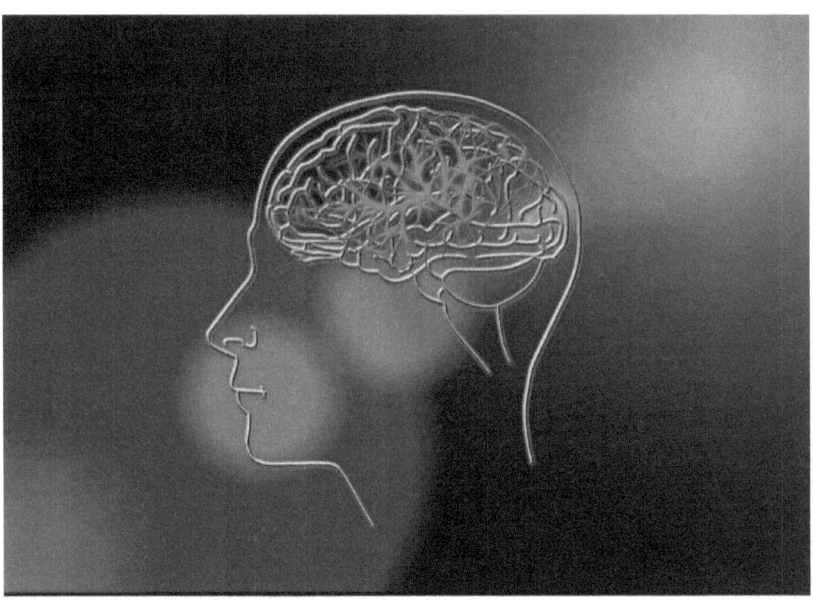

Minimize stroke-related PD risk by eating a balanced whole food diet, exercising daily, and getting 7-8 hours' sleep per night.

Take care of yourself and do what possible to avoid strokes, for they not only pose a health risk, but cause others such as Parkinson's disease or dementia.

Unhealthy diet

Eating an unhealthy diet is slow suicide on so many levels, but does it increase PD risks?

An unhealthy diet causes obesity, high blood pressure, and high blood sugar, three PD risk factors, but is there a direct link?

Often our worse enemy, we create a multitude of habits at work, home, or our social lives that destroy our health. We eat too large of servings of food loaded in sodium and preservatives, cooked the wrong way. We sit too many hours per day and get too little exercise.

A *Journal of Neurochemistry* study suggests obesity increases the risk of Parkinson's disease by inhibiting glucose and insulin[243].

Overeating the wrong foods can be as dangerous as being malnourished. If we do not provide the body and brain, the right combination of vegetables, fruits, fish, nuts, and berries, the brain and body suffer.

Vitamin deficiency

Vitamin D

Compared to our ancestors, modern humans avoid sunlight like vampires. Troglodytes got more sun, and they feared to leave the cave.

We know exceptions on the other extreme who cook their bodies medium-rare and continue until medium-well. They are the minority. We do not want this extreme anymore than not getting enough sun.

Unless we work in the sun, most of us do not get enough to absorb the Vitamin D our body and brains require to function and maintenance.

Studies suggest high levels of Vitamin D lower risks, while Vitamin D deficiencies increase the chances of Parkinson's disease.

What we know:

Vitamin D levels are low in both Parkinson's and dementia with Lewy body patients[244].

Get 15-20 minutes of sun per day and also consider taking a Vitamin D supplement. Vitamin D is vital for reducing Parkinson's disease and dementia with Lewy body risks, but also for your overall health.

Go for walks or other exercises in the sun where you combine exercise, Vitamin D gathering, fresh air, and the great outdoors.

V. BONUS SECTION

Whether diagnosed with dementia or preparing for a rainy day, there are basics everybody should consider.

This section focuses on steps dementia patients (all adults) should address, including forming a care team and understanding various therapy.

While written for dementia patients, I recommend every adult fulfill these tasks before you turn thirty. Waiting is our enemy for these two duties. Be prepared!

The section includes:

1. A starter to-do list for any adult diagnosed with a fatal disease such as dementia.
2. A care team plan.

JERRY BELLER HEALTH RESEARCH INSTITUTE

Chapter 17: Starter To-do List for Somebody and Family once Diagnosed with Dementia.

Dementia patients, loved ones, and family must address several matters early in the disease, including care, financial decisions, living quarters, Living Will, and Power of Attorney.

While you have full or most of your cognitive skills, take care of the listed priorities before diagnosis or when diagnosed. Please do not consider the items covered in this section a complete care list, but a start you tailor to your needs.

Fail to cross these items off the list while you maintain your facilities causes much regret for patients and loved ones.

Your life is your ship, and for now, you remain the captain. Plan how your ship faces the coming storm and, when you can no longer captain the ship yourself, have it already determined who takes over the helm.

Now remains your last best chance to have a substantial say in your future.

Care

Family, loved ones, and dementia patients must make difficult decisions concerning if somebody can become the primary volunteer caregiver. While dementia patients do not require 24/7 care in the early stage, it becomes necessary in the middle to late stages.

Nobody can get through dementia without others providing years of caregiving. While rare dementias kill in months, most dementia patients live for 5-20 years, with dementia growing progressively worse.

Diagnosed with dementia or in perfect health, we all must ask ourselves who would take care of us if dementia or another devastating disorder struck, requiring longterm caregiving.

Most families cannot afford professional caregiving, and the government will not help until towards the end, so family and loved ones must.

In an ideal world, we ask ourselves these tough questions and have a plan in place should something happen. This benefits not only those diagnosed with dementia but also the heroic voluntary caregivers who will see them to the end.

Financial Decisions

There are significant financial decisions to make, and earlier, the better.

Find out how much your insurance covers and the amount you must pay. A kinder world would not burden dementia patients, nor their loved ones, with overwhelming medical care costs.

In the United States and most countries in the world, the majority of dementia costs fall on families.

How Much Does Dementia Cost The Average Family?

With no urine or blood test for most dementia types, neurologists must rely on imaging and other expensive tests, often not to diagnose dementia but to rule out other neurological disorders.

Under the best scenario, related tests, doctor visits saddle the average patient with tens of thousands of dollars in deductibles by the time the neurological team diagnoses them with dementia. For some, such as dementia with Lewy bodies, it might run much higher as it can take up to eighteen months or longer before doctors make a correct diagnosis.

Our health system tells the average person: "Sorry, you have dementia. Oh, by the way, there's the bill."

Doctors, medical professionals, hospitals, drug companies, and others involved in treating dementia must make a living. Even when we factor out overcharging and profiteering, treating dementia would remain expensive.

The average American family's health insurance has deteriorated for years, the premiums growing too high, the deductibles unaffordable, and too many not worth the paper its written, much less the monthly premiums.

Authorities estimate the average cost per dementia patient is $341,840, with families expected to cover 70 percent.

Such a disease becomes a hardship for not only the patient but also their family. The demands, financial and otherwise, on voluntary caregivers often is devastating. Make difficult financial decisions early.

Financial costs vary from one dementia to another and the treatment plan.

Living Quarters

While most dementia patients maintain independence in stage one, at some point, they require help with daily tasks. Will somebody moves in with her or him? Does the patient move in with somebody else? Will it become necessary for him or her to move into an assisted living community in later stages? If so, what type?

The person diagnosed should gather loved ones and decide such matters in the beginning. Like somebody on a small island with a hurricane approaching, one must be diligent. While no man or woman can withstand such a storm, they still take precautions to protect themselves and their families.

In part because of financial considerations, most families care for the loved one in the home until symptoms grow critical. Whether a dementia patient ends up in a special needs living facility is not a matter of if, but at what point for those who have access.

No matter how much love, care, and attention a voluntary caregiver or loved ones provide a dementia patient, they are ill-equipped to provide for somebody in the disorder's final stretch.

Families without access do the best they can to provide comfort for the loved one but make no mistake, the patient and family benefit if a special needs facility takes over at some point.

Which type of facility depends on which dementia and symptoms. Some dementias cause more cognitive problems, while others greater affect motor skills, some visual, and a few dementias cause more language problems. In the end, many dementias are more alike than not, as the damage to the brain spreads to other areas. Still, depending on the symptoms, different care facilities might be better than others.

Ask your neurologist or local dementia organizations about local facilities trained for your particular type. Hopefully, you live at home and maintain a normal or semi-normal life for years, but have a facility selected when the end grows near.

Living Will

Not to be confused with a Last Will and Testament that distributes assets, a living will focus on medical decisions. NOLO defines a living will.

> *A living will – sometimes called a health care declaration -- is a document in which you describe the kind of health care you want to receive if you are incapacitated and cannot speak for yourself. It is often paired with a power of attorney for health care, in which you name an agent to make health care decisions on your behalf. Some states combine these two documents into one document called an 'advanced directive.'*

It is crucial to document the dementia patient's wishes while you maintain facilities to make such decisions.

Use the Living Will to direct physicians to follow your wishes on what care you receive now and in the future when you might not maintain your cognitive skills.

Specify end-of-life medical treatment.

NOLO recommends prioritizing life-prolonging medical care, food, and water if you become unconscious, and palliative care, which we soon address[245].

Distribute copies of your living will to loved ones, doctors, insurance providers, and all health care facilities.

Power of Attorney

The American Bar Association describes a power of attorney:

> *A power of attorney gives one or more persons the power to act on your behalf as your agent. The power may be limited to a particular activity, such as closing the sale of your home or be general in its application. The power may give temporary or permanent authority to act on your behalf. The power may take effect immediately, or only upon the occurrence of a future event, usually a determination that you are unable to act for yourself due to mental or physical disability. The latter is called a "springing" power of attorney. A power of attorney may be revoked, but most states require written notice of revocation to the person named to act for you[246].*

It is important to establish a medical power of attorney to empower a trusted loved one to make medical decisions when a patient becomes incapable. If you do not choose the right person, you can almost count on the wrong people making important decisions down the road.

If you're in early stages dementia and reading this, you likely can still think clearly, but this changes as the symptoms worsen. The only way to protect a dementia patient's wishes when they lose their cognitive decisionmaking is by naming a power of attorney in advance.

Once you name a power of attorney, cover some dos and don'ts. After all, you are trusting another person with your life. Like with your doctors, speak your mind while you can and let people know what you expect.

As NOLO pointed out, some states merge the living will and power of attorney into an advanced directive. Whether together or separate, I recommend all adults, and particularly those diagnosed with dementia draw up a medical living will and name a power of attorney.

The starter to-do list provides a starting point for dementia patients, families, and any adult.

Once diagnosed, both the person diagnosed and loved ones must unite and build your to-do list. Add whatever makes sense for you and your unique situation.

Let's next cover a few key members of a dementia care team.

Chapter 18: CARE TEAM

The National Institute on Aging recommends building a care team.

The team includes an art therapist, mental health counselor, occupational therapist, palliative care specialist, physical therapist, and a speech therapist[247].

Art therapist

The art therapist reduces stress by engaging the patient in music and other expressive arts.

Since dementia causes enormous anxiety and mood swings, art therapists use music and art to soothe patients and assist caregivers. Most everybody responds to music. Some pump our blood and makes us want to shake our bodies to the rhythm. Other music helps us focus and achieve maximum concentration.

Some music geared towards dementia patients relaxes and calms. Music is a godsend!

Art is not a task but a love affair. Some say within each of us is an artist starving to escape. Art therapists use music and art as a brilliant tool to treat dementia anxiety, attention decline, sleep problems, etc.

Mental health counselors

A neurological disorder, dementia attacks the brain and inhibits cognitive skills. Mental health counselors help patients and families plan for the future and cope with the shock, hurt, and pain resulting from the diagnosis.

Most individuals and families suffer chronic mental stress when doctors diagnose a member with dementia.

Find a mental health counselor trained in dementia.

Turn to their expertise and do not allow the neurological disorder to destroy the remaining quality of life for the patient, or respond as a family in a way where dementia destroys many lives by one sweeping event.

Occupational therapists

The occupational therapist helps patients bathe, dress, eat, and perform daily tasks.

We think of the routine daily tasks as second nature, and it is as long as the neurons, pathways, arteries, heart, and brain perform as normal. When suffering a stroke or neurological disorder like dementia, we quickly learn nothing is second nature anymore. Like a child, dementia patients often must relearn how to perform basic tasks.

Occupational therapists help patients remain independent and then semi-independent, as long as possible, extending the quality of life. An occupational therapist is instrumental in treating most dementias.

Palliative care specialist

The palliative care specialist minimizes symptoms from diagnosis to the end. You or a loved one need somebody who addresses symptoms as soon as they arise, so find a quality palliative care specialist.

They extend the quality of life and reduce suffering.

Physical therapists

Physical therapists help motors skills by leading patients through exercise.

Although dementia is known as a mental disorder, what affects the brain affects the body and vice versa. Find a physical therapist trained to work with your specific dementia.

If you've seen somebody suffering Parkinsonism or other neurological disorders affecting movement, you have an idea of the problems some dementias cause, even in the earliest stages.

A physical therapist helps maintain balance and strength, allowing a person to walk and move on their own. As dementia progresses, so does the physical therapist's importance.

Speech therapists

The speech therapist addresses speech and swallowing problems, issues present in early dementia symptoms for some types, and eventually becomes a problem for most dementias.

What is the value of verbalizing one's thoughts, understanding what a loved one says, and swallowing our food without choking or causing infection by sending it down the wrong pipe?

These are issues speech therapists excel. The ones I've observed are passionate about helping people retrain the mind to overcome aphasia and swallowing problems.

Find a speech (and other types of) therapist trained in treating your specific type of dementia. These different listed therapists can minimize the long nightmare following a dementia diagnosis.

Chapter 19: LETTER TO CONGRESS

DEAR U.S. CONGRESS, NATIONS OF THE WORLD, & WEALTHY HUMANS

We call on the United States and the governments of the world to spend less on war and walls and more on Alzheimer's and dementia research.

If aliens were attacking us from another planet, I presume the nations of the world would unite against a common enemy. That is what I propose now.

The enemy I refer to does not come from another planet but threatens humans no less. Alzheimer's and dementia strike an American every 68 seconds and somebody worldwide every 30 seconds.

The nations of the world can save millions of lives and billions of dollars.

We need necessary funding to:

1. Discover the exact cause (s) of Alzheimer's and other dementias.
2. Develop accurate testing for Alzheimer's and other dementias.
3. Develop a vaccine to wipe out Alzheimer's and other dementias like we did polio.

Alzheimer's and dementia grow at a rate that will destroy the economies of most countries if we do not become more proactive.

We can save trillions of dollars for future generations if we invest now in discovering the exact cause (s), a vaccine to prevent it from happening, and other steps to defeat this horrifying disease.

Alzheimer's and other dementias threaten every family in all nations.

We can do little for those with late-stage dementia, but the proposed steps might save millions of lives and trillions of dollars by diagnosing the different dementias early and treating them before they do significant damage.

Beller Health calls on politicians, corporations, and wealthy individuals to step forward to help win the war against dementia.

CONCLUSION

Thank you for reading this book. We covered a good amount of material.

Dementia is a cruel neurological disorder that robs people of their personalities, executive skills, memories, talents, language, voice, motor capabilities, and all that makes us individual humans.

Dementia Spares No Demographic

Dementia's reputation is known as an old folk's disease but strikes people all ages. Most dementia is not genetic, although certain types such as Huntington's disease are 100% familial.

Most Dementia is Incurable

Most dementia is incurable, but—if caught early enough—neurosurgeons can treat and sometimes reverse normal pressure hydrocephalus.

Dementia Prevalence

The first section focused on dementia as a general category. We learned 850,000 people in the UK have dementia, compared to 5.8 Americans and 50 million people worldwide.

Dementia Categories

We divided the 19 dementias into six categories:

- Lewy Body/Parkinsonism related dementias
- Alzheimer's related dementias
- Frontotemporal lobar degeneration related dementias

- Primary progressive aphasia related dementias
- Vascular dementias
- Other dementias

19 Dementia Types
Lewy Body/Parkinsonism Related Dementias

1. *Dementia with Lewy Bodies*
2. *Parkinson's Disease Dementia*
3. Corticobasal Syndrome

Alzheimer's Related Dementias

4. Typical Alzheimer's Disease
5. *Posterior Cortical Atrophy*
6. *Down Syndrome with Alzheimer's*
7. *Limbic-predominant Age-related TDP-43 Encephalopathy (LATE)*
8. Early-onset Alzheimer's

Frontotemporal Lobar Degeneration Related Dementias

9. *Behavioral Variant Frontotemporal Dementia*
10. Progressive Supranuclear Palsy

Primary Progressive Aphasia Related Dementias

11. *Nonfluent Primary Progressive Aphasia (nfvPPA)*
12. Logopenic Progressive Aphasia (LPA)

Vascular Dementia

13. *Cortical Vascular Dementia*
14. *Binswanger Disease*

Other Dementias

15. *Normal Pressure Hydrocephalus*
16. *Huntington's Disease*
17. *Korsakoff Syndrome*
18. *Creutzfeldt-Jakob Disease*
19. Amyotrophic Lateral Sclerosis

Once we defined and discussed dementia, and listed the 19 types, we shifted the conversation to the Lewy body and Parkinsonism related dementias.

We learned dementia with Lewy bodies (DLB), and Parkinson's disease dementia (PDD) are the same disorder, but take opposite paths.

Early dementia with Lewy bodies' symptoms is more dementia-oriented, while Parkinson's symptoms develop later. PDD begins with Parkinson's disease and evolves into dementia. At some point, they become the same neurological disorder suffering both Parkinson's and dementia.

We learned Corticobasal syndrome (CS) is a Parkinson's plus disorder, meaning it exhibits most Parkinson's symptoms and some additional ones unique to CS.

We covered prevalence, cause, symptoms, stages, and risk factors for all three subtypes.

THE END

Of

LEWY BODY & PARKINSONISM DEMENTIAS

THANK YOU FOR READING

Thank you for reading the entire book. While this is not a literary work to enjoy, I hope you gained useful knowledge of posterior cortical atrophy.

If you benefitted from this book, please take a moment to share your thoughts in a review. Reader reviews help other readers make educated decisions about this book before purchasing.

Book Review link for Lewy Body & Parkinsonism Dementias

or

https://www.amazon.com/dp/B07XLMW877

Look for annual updates to my health books, as I follow new studies and add any helpful information I find. Health and fitness are top priorities, and the heart and brain are my specialties.

I hope you develop the habits suggested in this book. Good luck on your health journey. Live long and prosper, my friend.

All the best,
Jerry Beller & Beller Health

BELLER HEALTH BOOKS

Beller Health Research Institute specializes in the heart and brain, and published the following Jerry Beller book series:

- Arrhythmia Series
- Vascular Disease Series
- 2020 Dementia Overview Series
- 19 Dementia Types Series

Please continue to view the books in each series.

Dementia Types, Symptoms, Stages, & Risk Factors Series

This book series is the first to cover each of the 19 primary dementia types.

1. *Dementia with Lewy Bodies*
2. *Parkinson's Disease Dementia*
3. Corticobasal Syndrome
4. Typical Alzheimer's Disease
5. *Posterior Cortical Atrophy*
6. *Down Syndrome with Alzheimer's*
7. *Limbic-predominant Age-related TDP-43 Encephalopathy (LATE)*
8. Early-onset Alzheimer's
9. *Behavioral Variant Frontotemporal Dementia*
10. Progressive Supranuclear Palsy
11. *Nonfluent Primary Progressive Aphasia*
12. Logopenic Progressive Aphasia
13. *Cortical Vascular Dementia*
14. *Binswanger Disease*
15. *Normal Pressure Hydrocephalus*
16. *Huntington's Disease*
17. *Korsakoff Syndrome*
18. *Creutzfeldt-Jakob Disease*
19. Amyotrophic Lateral Sclerosis

2020 Dementia Overview Series

Whereas in the *Dementia Types, Symptoms, Stages, and Risk Factors* series, each book covers a different dementia type, this series focuses on groups of dementias.

1. Dementia Types, Symptoms, & Stages
2. *Lewy Body/Parkinsonism Dementias*
3. *Vascular Dementia*
4. *Frontotemporal Dementia (FTD)*
5. Alzheimer's Related Dementias
6. *Prevent or Slow Dementia*

Other Beller Health Books

You can view or purchase all Beller Health Books on Amazon at the following web address:

https://amzn.to/2TpDr8e

ABOUT THE AUTHOR

Jerry Beller is the lead author and researcher at Beller Medical Research Institute. Beller distinguished himself three times in the medical world by being the first to write and publish books on particular dementia fields.

He wrote the first book covering all 15 primary dementia types, which he since expanded to cover nineteen. Beller followed this accomplishment by writing a book on each dementia type. He broke medical ground a third time when he published the first book on the new dementia category LATE.

When the world struggled to grasp the difference between Alzheimer's disease and China, Beller explained:

Alzheimer's is only one dementia, much like China is only one country in Asia. Just as we do not want to ignore the other countries in Asia because China is the largest, nor do we want to ignore the less prevalent dementia types.

Despite his accomplishments, he remains humble. "Until we win the dementia war, I've no reason to celebrate," Beller said. "If we win the war during my lifetime, I will celebrate with a few hundred brothers and sisters around the world who share my passion. Until then, we have too much work left to worry about accolades and legacies."

When not researching dementia, Jerry enjoys life with his wife of thirty-plus years, Nicola, and their two children.

Visit Jerry Beller at:

https://bellerhealth.com

1 'What Is Dementia?', Alzheimer's Disease and Dementia <https://alz.org/alzheimers-dementia/what-is-dementia> [accessed 18 September 2019].

2 'What Is Dementia? Symptoms, Types, and Diagnosis', National Institute on Aging <https://www.nia.nih.gov/health/what-dementia-symptoms-types-and-diagnosis> [accessed 18 September 2019].

[3] 'What Is Dementia?', *Alzheimer's Society* <https://www.alzheimers.org.uk/about-dementia/types-dementia/what-dementia> [accessed 18 September 2019].

[4] 'Dementia' <https://www.who.int/news-room/fact-sheets/detail/dementia> [accessed 18 September 2019].

[5] 'Risk Factors' <https://stanfordhealthcare.org/medical-conditions/brain-and-nerves/dementia/risk-factors.html> [accessed 20 September 2019].

[6] W. M. van der Flier and P. Scheltens, 'Epidemiology and Risk Factors of Dementia', *Journal of Neurology, Neurosurgery & Psychiatry*, 76.suppl 5 (2005), v2–7 <https://doi.org/10.1136/jnnp.2005.082867>.

[7] Kent Allen, 'Dementia Rates to Grow for African Americans, Hispanics', *AARP* <http://www.aarp.org/health/dementia/info-2018/dementia-alzheimer-cases-grow-nonwhites.html> [accessed 20 September 2019].

[8] Elizabeth Rose Mayeda and others, 'Inequalities in Dementia Incidence between Six Racial and Ethnic Groups over 14 Years', *Alzheimer's & Dementia: The Journal of the Alzheimer's Association*, 12.3 (2016), 216–24 <https://doi.org/10.1016/j.jalz.2015.12.007>.

[9] 'African Americans at Higher Dementia Risk than Other Racial Groups', *Reuters*, 10 March 2016 <https://www.reuters.com/article/us-health-dementia-race-u-s-idUSKCN0WC2X5> [accessed 20 September 2019].

[10] Steve Ford, 'Likelihood of Dementia "Higher among Black Ethnic Groups"', *Nursing Times*, 2018 <https://www.nursingtimes.net/news/research-and-innovation/likelihood-of-dementia-higher-among-black-ethnic-groups-08-08-2018/> [accessed 21 September 2019].

[11] 'Dementia' <https://www.who.int/news-room/fact-sheets/detail/dementia> [accessed 21 September 2019].

189

[12] 'Women and Alzheimer's', *Alzheimer's Disease and Dementia* <https://alz.org/alzheimers-dementia/what-is-alzheimers/women-and-alzheimer-s> [accessed 21 September 2019].

[13] 'Dementia Facts', *Dementia Consortium* <https://www.dementiaconsortium.org/dementia-facts/> [accessed 21 September 2019].

[14] 'Dementia' <https://www.who.int/news-room/fact-sheets/detail/dementia> [accessed 21 September 2019].

[15] 'Why Is Dementia Different for Women?', *Alzheimer's Society* <https://www.alzheimers.org.uk/blog/why-dementia-different-women> [accessed 21 September 2019].

[16] Jessica L. Podcasy and C. Neill Epperson, 'Considering Sex and Gender in Alzheimer Disease and Other Dementias', *Dialogues in Clinical Neuroscience*, 18.4 (2016), 437–46 <https://www.ncbi.nlm.nih.gov/pmc/articles/PMC5286729/> [accessed 21 September 2019].

[17] 'WHO | Life Expectancy', *WHO* <http://www.who.int/gho/mortality_burden_disease/life_tables/situation_trends_text/en/> [accessed 21 September 2019].

[18] 'Products - Data Briefs - Number 328 - November 2018', 2019 <https://www.cdc.gov/nchs/products/databriefs/db328.htm> [accessed 21 September 2019].

[19] Jacqui Thornton, 'WHO Report Shows That Women Outlive Men Worldwide', *BMJ*, 365 (2019), l1631 <https://doi.org/10.1136/bmj.l1631>.

[20] 'Why Do Women Live Longer Than Men?', *Time* <https://time.com/5538099/why-do-women-live-longer-than-men/> [accessed 21 September 2019].

[21] 'Dementia' <https://www.who.int/news-room/fact-sheets/detail/dementia> [accessed 20 September 2019].

[22] 'Alzheimer's Disease: Facts & Figures', *BrightFocus Foundation*, 2015 <https://www.brightfocus.org/alzheimers/article/alzheimers-disease-facts-figures> [accessed 4 September 2019].

[23] 'Facts for the Media', *Alzheimer's Society* <https://www.alzheimers.org.uk/about-us/news-and-media/facts-media> [accessed 20 September 2019].

[24] 'Countries With The Highest Rates Of Deaths From Dementia',

WorldAtlas <https://www.worldatlas.com/articles/countries-with-the-highest-rates-of-deaths-from-dementia.html> [accessed 20 September 2019].

[25] 'World Alzheimer Report 2018 - The State of the Art of Dementia Research: New Frontiers', *NEW FRONTIERS*, 48.

[26] 'ALZHEIMERS/DEMENTIA DEATH RATE BY COUNTRY', *World Life Expectancy* <https://www.worldlifeexpectancy.com/cause-of-death/alzheimers-dementia/by-country/> [accessed 24 September 2019].

[27] 'Alzheimer Europe - Research - European Collaboration on Dementia - Cost of Dementia - Regional/National Cost of Illness Estimates' <https://www.alzheimer-europe.org/Research/European-Collaboration-on-Dementia/Cost-of-dementia/Regional-National-cost-of-illness-estimates> [accessed 26 September 2019].

[28] 'Publications | NATSEM' <https://www.natsem.canberra.edu.au/publications/?publication=economic-cost-of-dementia-in-australia-2016-2056> [accessed 22 September 2019].

[29] 'Dementia UK Report', *Alzheimer's Society* <https://www.alzheimers.org.uk/about-us/policy-and-influencing/dementia-uk-report> [accessed 22 September 2019].

[30] 'Dementia Statistics – U.S. & Worldwide Stats', *BrainTest*, 2015 <https://braintest.com/dementia-stats-u-s-worldwide/> [accessed 23 September 2019].

[31] 'Newsroom | Northwestern Mutual - 2018 C.A.R.E. Study', *Newsroom | Northwestern Mutual* <https://news.northwesternmutual.com/2018-care-study> [accessed 22 September 2019].

[32] 'ALZHEIMERS/DEMENTIA DEATH RATE BY COUNTRY'.

[33] 'Alzheimer Europe - Research - European Collaboration on Dementia - Cost of Dementia - Regional/National Cost of Illness Estimates'.

[34] 'Publications | NATSEM'.

[35] 'Dementia UK Report'.

[36] 'Dementia Statistics – U.S. & Worldwide Stats'.

[37] 'Friedrich Heinrich Lewy Body Dementia Lewey Frederic Shaking Palsy Paralysis Agitans Parkinson Hans Förstl' <http://www2.psykl.med.tum.de/geschichte_history/lewy1991.html> [accessed 6 January 2019].

[38] Bernd Holdorff, 'Friedrich Heinrich Lewy (1885-1950) and His Work', *Journal of the History of the Neurosciences*, 11.1 (2002), 19–28 <https://doi.org/10.1076/jhin.11.1.19.9106>.

[39] Suraj Rajan, *English: Photomicrograph of Regions of Substantia Nigra in a Parkinson's Patient Showing Lewy Bodies and Lewy Neurites in Various Magnifications. Top Panels Show a 60-Times Magnification of the Alpha Synuclein Intraneuronal Inclusions Aggregated to Form Lewy Bodies. The Bottom Panels Are 20 × Magnification Images That Show Strand-like Lewy Neurites and Rounded Lewy Bodies of Various Sizes. Neuromelanin Laden Cells of the Substantia Nigra Are Visible in the Background. Stains Used: Mouse Monoclonal Alpha-Synuclein Antibody; Counterstained with Mayer's Haematoxylin.*, 2012, Own work <https://commons.wikimedia.org/wiki/File:Lewy_bodies_(alpha_synuclein_inclusions).svg> [accessed 23 April 2019].

[40] 'Lewy Body Dementia - Symptoms and Causes - Mayo Clinic' <https://www.mayoclinic.org/diseases-conditions/lewy-body-dementia/symptoms-causes/syc-20352025> [accessed 18 February 2018].

[41] 'What Is LBD? | Lewy Body Dementia Association' <https://www.lbda.org/category/3437/what-is-lbd.htm> [accessed 18 February 2018].

[42] 'Parkinson's Disease Dementia', *Memory and Aging Center* <https://memory.ucsf.edu/parkinson-disease-dementia> [accessed 24 April 2019].

[43] Rajan.

[44] 'A New Insight into Parkinson's Disease Protein | UC San Francisco', *A New Insight into Parkinson's Disease Protein | UC San Francisco* <https://www.ucsf.edu/news/2017/07/407866/new-insight-parkinsons-disease-protein> [accessed 24 April 2019].

[45] 'Chapter 11: The Cerebral Cortex' <https://www.dartmouth.edu/~rswenson/NeuroSci/chapter_11.html> [accessed 24 April 2019].

[46] 'Human Brain', *Wikipedia*, 2019 <https://en.wikipedia.org/w/index.php?title=Human_brain&oldid=893696243> [accessed 24 April 2019].

[47] T. Huff and S. C. Dulebohn, 'Neuroanatomy, Visual Cortex', 2018 <http://europepmc.org/abstract/med/29494110> [accessed 24 April 2019].

[48] 'ASSOCIATION CORTEX' <http://www.indiana.edu/~p1013447/dictionary/assn_cor.htm> [accessed 24 April 2019].

[49] 'Know Your Brain: Primary Somatosensory Cortex — Neuroscientifically

Challenged' <https://neuroscientificallychallenged.com/blog/know-your-brain-primary-somatosensory-cortex> [accessed 24 April 2019].

⁵⁰ Simon B. Eickhoff and others, 'Anatomical and Functional Connectivity of Cytoarchitectonic Areas within the Human Parietal Operculum', *The Journal of Neuroscience: The Official Journal of the Society for Neuroscience*, 30.18 (2010), 6409–21 <https://doi.org/10.1523/JNEUROSCI.5664-09.2010>.

⁵¹ Fritzie I. Arce-McShane and others, 'Primary Motor and Sensory Cortical Areas Communicate via Spatiotemporally Coordinated Networks at Multiple Frequencies', *Proceedings of the National Academy of Sciences of the United States of America*, 113.18 (2016), 5083–88 <https://doi.org/10.1073/pnas.1600788113>.

⁵² *Neuroscience*, 2nd edn (Sinauer Associates, 2001).

⁵³ Lutz Jäncke, Marcus Cheetham, and Thomas Baumgartner, 'Virtual Reality and the Role of the Prefrontal Cortex in Adults and Children.', *Frontiers in Neuroscience*, 3 (2009) <https://doi.org/10.3389/neuro.01.006.2009>.

⁵⁴ 'Lewy Body Dementias', *Memory and Aging Center* <https://memory.ucsf.edu/lewy-body-dementias> [accessed 24 April 2019].

⁵⁵ 'Dementia with Lewy Bodies (DLB) | Johns Hopkins Medicine' <https://www.hopkinsmedicine.org/health/conditions-and-diseases/dementia/dementia-with-lewy-bodies> [accessed 24 April 2019].

⁵⁶ 'What Is LBD? | Lewy Body Dementia Association' <https://www.lbda.org/go/what-lbd-0> [accessed 24 April 2019].

⁵⁷ '10 Things You Should Know about LBD | Lewy Body Dementia Association' <https://www.lbda.org/go/10-things-you-should-know-about-lbd> [accessed 24 April 2019].

⁵⁸ Yoshio Tsuboi and Dennis W. Dickson, 'Dementia with Lewy Bodies and Parkinson's Disease with Dementia: Are They Different?', *Parkinsonism & Related Disorders*, 11 Suppl 1 (2005), S47-51 <https://doi.org/10.1016/j.parkreldis.2004.10.014>.

⁵⁹ 'The LBD Spectrum | Lewy Body Dementia Association' <https://www.lbda.org/content/lbd-spectrum> [accessed 22 February 2018].

⁶⁰ 'Dementia with Lewy Bodies (DLB)', *Cedars-Sinai* <https://www.cedars-sinai.org/health-library/diseases-and-conditions/d/dementia-with-lewy-bodies-dlb.html> [accessed 24 April 2019].

⁶¹ 'Dementia with Lewy Bodies Symptoms| Signs, Symptoms, & Diagnosis', *Dementia* <//www.alz.org/dementia/dementia-with-lewy-bodies-symptoms.asp> [accessed 18 February 2018].

⁶² James E. Galvin and others, 'LEWY BODY DEMENTIA: THE

CAREGIVER EXPERIENCE OF CLINICAL CARE', *Parkinsonism & Related Disorders*, 16.6 (2010), 388–92 <https://doi.org/10.1016/j.parkreldis.2010.03.007>.

[63] '10 Things You Need to Know about Lewy Body Dementia | Lewy Body Dementia Association' <https://www.lbda.org/content/10-things-you-need-know-about-lewy-body-dementia> [accessed 18 February 2018].

[64] Allan Ajifo, *BY ALLAN AJIFO [CC BY 2.0 (HTTP://CREATIVECOMMONS.ORG/LICENSES/BY/2.0)], VIA WIKIMEDIA COMMONS*, 2009, https://www.flickr.com/photos/125992663@N02/14414604077/ <https://commons.wikimedia.org/wiki/File:Brain_parts.jpg> [accessed 18 February 2018].

[65] 'Parkinson's Disease Statistics', *Parkinson's News Today* <https://parkinsonsnewstoday.com/parkinsons-disease-statistics/> [accessed 25 April 2019].

[66] 'What Is Parkinson's?', *Parkinson's Foundation*, 2015 <https://parkinson.org/understanding-parkinsons/what-is-parkinsons> [accessed 25 April 2019].

[67] 'What Is Parkinson's? | American Parkinson Disease Assoc.', *APDA* <https://www.apdaparkinson.org/what-is-parkinsons/> [accessed 25 April 2019].

[68] 'Parkinson's Foundation: Better Lives. Together.' <https://www.parkinson.org/Understanding-Parkinsons/Statistics> [accessed 25 April 2019].

[69] 'Understanding Parkinson's and Parkinson's Dementia', *Healthline*, 2016 <https://www.healthline.com/health/parkinsons/parkinsons-dementia> [accessed 25 April 2019].

[70] H. Ling and others, 'Does Corticobasal Degeneration Exist? A Clinicopathological Re-Evaluation', *Brain*, 133.7 (2010), 2045–57 <https://doi.org/10.1093/brain/awq123>.

[71] W. R. Gibb, P. J. Luthert, and C. D. Marsden, 'Corticobasal Degeneration', *Brain: A Journal of Neurology*, 112 (Pt 5) (1989), 1171–92 <https://doi.org/10.1093/brain/112.5.1171>.

[72] 'Corticobasal Syndrome (CBS)', *Baylor College of Medicine* <https://www.bcm.edu/healthcare/care-centers/parkinsons/conditions/corticobasal-syndrome> [accessed 4 December 2019].

[73] Andreea L. Seritan and others, 'Functional Imaging as a Window to Dementia: Corticobasal Degeneration', *The Journal of Neuropsychiatry and Clinical Neurosciences*, 16.4 (2004), 393–99

<https://doi.org/10.1176/jnp.16.4.393>.

74 'Corticobasal Degeneration', *NORD (National Organization for Rare Disorders)* <https://rarediseases.org/rare-diseases/corticobasal-degeneration/> [accessed 6 December 2019].

75 'Corticobasal Syndrome', *Memory and Aging Center* <https://memory.ucsf.edu/dementia/corticobasal-syndrome> [accessed 4 December 2019].

76 'Gait Abnormalities', *Stanford Medicine 25* <https://stanfordmedicine25.stanford.edu/the25/gait.html> [accessed 24 April 2019].

77 James E. Galvin, 'Improving the Clinical Detection of Lewy Body Dementia with the Lewy Body Composite Risk Score', *Alzheimer's & Dementia: Diagnosis, Assessment & Disease Monitoring*, 1.3 (2015), 316–24 <https://doi.org/10.1016/j.dadm.2015.05.004>.

78 'Lewy Body Dementia - Symptoms and Causes - Mayo Clinic'.

79 'Dementia Symptoms: Illusions, Hallucinations and Delusions' <https://healthblog.uofmhealth.org/brain-health/illusions-hallucinations-and-delusions-how-to-spot-dementia-symptoms> [accessed 18 February 2018].

80 'Dementia with Lewy Bodies Symptoms - Six Signs of the Disease | Health | Life & Style | Express.Co.Uk' <https://www.express.co.uk/life-style/health/809643/dementia-lewy-bodies-symptoms-vascular-alzheimers> [accessed 18 February 2018].

81 'Lewy Body Dementia' <https://patient.info/health/memory-loss-and-dementia/lewy-body-dementia> [accessed 18 February 2018].

82 Carolyn Steber, 'Signs Your Brain Fog Is More Serious Than You Might Think', *Bustle* <https://www.bustle.com/p/11-signs-your-brain-might-be-slowing-down-earlier-than-it-should-80166> [accessed 18 February 2018].

83 'Lewy Body Dementia - Symptoms and Causes - Mayo Clinic'.

84 'How Lewy Body Dementia Contributes to Depression' <https://www.alzheimers.net/11-21-14-lewy-body-depression-hallucinations/> [accessed 18 February 2018].

85 'What Is Lewy Body Dementia?', *WebMD* <https://www.webmd.com/alzheimers/guide/dementia-lewy-bodies> [accessed 18 February 2018].

86 'How Lewy Body Dementia Contributes to Depression'.

87 'Symptoms | Lewy Body Dementia Association' <https://www.lbda.org/content/symptoms> [accessed 18 February 2018].

88 'News You Can Use: Fall Prevention Tips | Lewy Body Dementia Association' <https://www.lbda.org/content/news-you-can-use-fall-prevention-tips> [accessed 18 February 2018].

89 'ComparisonofdementiawithLewybidoesto.Pdf' <http://www.cumc.columbia.edu/dept/sergievsky/pdfs/Comparisonofdementiaw ithLewybidoesto.pdf> [accessed 18 February 2018].

90 'Lewy Body Dementia: Information for Patients, Families, and Professionals | Lewy Body Dementia Association' <https://www.lbda.org/content/lewy-body-dementia-information-patients-families-and-professionals> [accessed 18 February 2018].

91 'Reduce Dementia-Related Swallowing Problems. Avoid Aspiration. - Lewy Body Dementia' <http://www.lewybodydementia.ca/solve-swallowing-problems-and-avoid-aspiration-in-dementia/> [accessed 18 February 2018].

92 'ALZ026-DLB-0116-0118_FEB-2016_WEB.Pdf' <https://www.alzheimersresearchuk.org/wp-content/uploads/2015/02/ALZ026-DLB-0116-0118_FEB-2016_WEB.pdf> [accessed 18 February 2018].

93 'Living Well with Lewy Body Dementia and Comorbidities : Dementia and Chest Infections', *Living Well with Lewy Body Dementia and Comorbidities*, 2013 <http://ken-kenc2.blogspot.com/2013/11/dementia-and-chest-infections.html> [accessed 18 February 2018].

94 'Lewy Body Dementia - Symptoms and Causes', *Mayo Clinic* <https://www.mayoclinic.org/diseases-conditions/lewy-body-dementia/symptoms-causes/syc-20352025> [accessed 15 November 2019].

95 'What Is Lewy Body Dementia?', *National Institute on Aging* <https://www.nia.nih.gov/health/what-lewy-body-dementia> [accessed 15 November 2019].

96 '10 Things You Should Know about LBD | Lewy Body Dementia Association' <https://www.lbda.org/go/10-things-you-should-know-about-lbd> [accessed 15 November 2019].

97 'Dementia with Lewy Bodies - Symptoms', *Nhs.Uk*, 2018 <https://www.nhs.uk/conditions/dementia-with-lewy-bodies/symptoms/> [accessed 15 November 2019].

98 'Gait Abnormalities'.

99 'Dementia' <https://www.who.int/news-room/fact-sheets/detail/dementia> [accessed 13 December 2018].

100 'Parkinsons_Disease' <http://www.thepi.org/faq/parkinsons-disease>

[accessed 24 April 2019].

[101] 'Non-Movement Symptoms', *Parkinson's Foundation*, 2017 <https://parkinson.org/Understanding-Parkinsons/Non-Movement-Symptoms> [accessed 25 April 2019].

[102] K. Ray Chaudhuri, Daniel G. Healy, and Anthony HV Schapira, 'Non-Motor Symptoms of Parkinson's Disease: Diagnosis and Management', *The Lancet Neurology*, 5.3 (2006), 235–45 <https://doi.org/10.1016/S1474-4422(06)70373-8>.

[103] 'Cognitive Impairment in Parkinson's Disease', *Parkinson's News Today* <https://parkinsonsnewstoday.com/parkinsons-disease-symptoms/non-motor/cognitive-impairment/> [accessed 17 November 2019].

[104] European Parkinson's Disease Association, 'Motor Symptoms' <http://www.epda.eu.com/about-parkinsons/symptoms/motor-symptoms/> [accessed 25 April 2019].

[105] 'Movement Symptoms', *Parkinson's Foundation*, 2017 <https://parkinson.org/Understanding-Parkinsons/Movement-Symptoms> [accessed 25 April 2019].

[106] 'The LBD Spectrum | Lewy Body Dementia Association' <https://www.lbda.org/go/lbd-spectrum> [accessed 25 April 2019].

[107] Alexander Pantelyat and others, 'Acalculia in Autopsy-Proven Corticobasal Degeneration', *Neurology*, 76.7 0 2 (2011), S61–63 <https://doi.org/10.1212/WNL.0b013e31820c34ca>.

[108] 'What Is Parkinson's & What Does It Do' <https://www.parkinsonswa.org.au/what-is-parkinsons/> [accessed 6 December 2019].

[109] Jonathan Graff-Radford and others, 'The Alien Limb Phenomenon', *Journal of Neurology*, 260.7 (2013), 1880–88 <https://doi.org/10.1007/s00415-013-6898-y>.

[110] 'Apraxia', *NORD (National Organization for Rare Disorders)* <https://rarediseases.org/rare-diseases/apraxia/> [accessed 6 December 2019].

[111] 'Limb Apraxia', *American Speech-Language-Hearing Association* <https://www.asha.org/Glossary/Limb-Apraxia/> [accessed 6 December 2019].

[112] A. Berardelli and others, 'Pathophysiology of Bradykinesia in Parkinson's Disease', *Brain*, 124.11 (2001), 2131–46 <https://doi.org/10.1093/brain/124.11.2131>.

113 European Parkinson's Disease Association, 'Bradykinesia' <https://www.epda.eu.com/about-parkinsons/symptoms/motor-symptoms/bradykinesia/> [accessed 6 December 2019].

114 'What Is Dystonia? | Dystonia Medical Research Foundation' <https://dystonia-foundation.org/what-is-dystonia/> [accessed 6 December 2019].

115 'Dystonia – Classifications, Symptoms and Treatment' <https://www.aans.org/> [accessed 6 December 2019].

116 Theodore P. Parthimos and Kleopatra H. Schulpis, 'The Significant Characteristics of Corticobasal Syndrome', *Annals of Research Hospitals*, 3.0 (2019) <http://arh.amegroups.com/article/view/4676> [accessed 6 December 2019].

117 'WEBINAR-HANDOUT-2015-LBD-Fact-Sheet-A.Pdf' <http://www.nadsa.org/wp-content/uploads/2015/06/WEBINAR-HANDOUT-2015-LBD-Fact-Sheet-A.pdf> [accessed 24 April 2019].

118 Galvin.

119 'Characteristics of Facial Expression Recognition Ability in Patients with Lewy Body Disease | Environmental Health and Preventive Medicine | Full Text' <https://environhealthprevmed.biomedcentral.com/articles/10.1186/s12199-018-0723-2> [accessed 24 April 2019].

120 'Symptoms', *The Lewy Body Society* <https://www.lewybody.org/about-lbd/symptoms/> [accessed 24 April 2019].

121 'Personality Changes May Help Detect Form Of Dementia', *ScienceDaily* <https://www.sciencedaily.com/releases/2007/05/070528160810.htm> [accessed 24 April 2019].

122 Ray-Chang Tzeng and others, 'Delusions in Patients with Dementia with Lewy Bodies and the Associated Factors', *Behavioural Neurology*, 2018 (2018), 6707291 <https://doi.org/10.1155/2018/6707291>.

123 'Dementia with Lewy Bodies', *Neurology* <http://www.columbianeurology.org/neurology/staywell/document.php> [accessed 15 November 2019].

124 'Lewy Body Dementia Treatment & Management: Approach Considerations', 2019 <https://emedicine.medscape.com/article/1135041-treatment> [accessed 15 November 2019].

125 'The Progression of Dementia with Lewy Bodies', *Alzheimer's Society* <https://www.alzheimers.org.uk/about-dementia/symptoms-and-diagnosis/how-

dementia-progresses/progression-dementia-lewy-bodies> [accessed 24 April 2019].

126 'UCSF Weill Institute for Neurosciences', *UCSF Neurosciences* <https://weill.ucsf.edu/ucsf-weill-institute-neurosciences> [accessed 24 April 2019].

127 'UCSF_LBD_Providers_7-13-17.Pdf' <https://memory.ucsf.edu/sites/memory.ucsf.edu/files/wysiwyg/UCSF_LBD_Pr oviders_7-13-17.pdf> [accessed 24 April 2019].

128 'In Dementia with Lewy Bodies, Braak Stage Determines Phenotype, Not Lewy Body Distribution | Neurology' <https://n.neurology.org/content/dementia-lewy-bodies-braak-stage-determines-phenotype-not-lewy-body-distribution-0> [accessed 24 April 2019].

129 'UCSF Weill Institute for Neurosciences'.

130 Pietro Tiraboschi and others, 'What Best Differentiates Lewy Body from Alzheimer's Disease in Early-Stage Dementia?', *Brain*, 129.3 (2006), 729–35 <https://doi.org/10.1093/brain/awh725>.

131 'Lewy Body Dementia - Symptoms and Causes - Mayo Clinic' <https://www.mayoclinic.org/diseases-conditions/lewy-body-dementia/symptoms-causes/syc-20352025> [accessed 24 April 2019].

132 'Stages or Phases of Lewy Body Dementia', *Lewy Body Dementia* <http://www.lewybodydementia.ca/lewy-body-dementia-phases-and-stages/> [accessed 24 April 2019].

133 Paul C. Donaghy and Ian G. McKeith, 'The Clinical Characteristics of Dementia with Lewy Bodies and a Consideration of Prodromal Diagnosis', *Alzheimer's Research & Therapy*, 6.4 (2014), 46 <https://doi.org/10.1186/alzrt274>.

134 'DLB Early Stages – Rare Dementia Support' <http://www.raredementiasupport.org/lewy-body-dementia/dlb-early-stages/> [accessed 24 April 2019].

135 Mariya Petrova and others, 'Clinical and Neuropsychological Differences between Mild Parkinson's Disease Dementia and Dementia with Lewy Bodies', *Dementia and Geriatric Cognitive Disorders Extra*, 5.2 (2015), 212–20 <https://doi.org/10.1159/000375363>.

136 Ian G Mckeith, 'DEMENTIA WITH LEWY BODIES', 16.

137 'Johntroj.Pdf' <https://www.alz.washington.edu/NONMEMBER/FALL08/johntroj.pdf> [accessed 24 April 2019].

138 'The Neuropathologic Substrate of Parkinson Disease Dementia' <https://www.e-jmd.org/journal/view.php?doi=10.14802/jmd.09001> [accessed

199

24 April 2019].

139 'MDS Rating Scales'
<https://www.movementdisorders.org/MDS/Education/Rating-Scales.htm>
[accessed 25 April 2019].

140 'Unified Parkinson's Disease Rating Scale (UPDRS) | Parkinson's UK'
<https://www.parkinsons.org.uk/professionals/resources/unified-parkinsons-disease-rating-scale-updrs> [accessed 25 April 2019].

141 'What Is Parkinson's Disease Dyskinesia?', *Davis Phinney Foundation*, 2018
<https://www.davisphinneyfoundation.org/blog/what-is-parkinsons-disease-dyskinesia/> [accessed 25 April 2019].

142 American Speech-Language-Hearing Association (ASHA), 'Definitions of Communication Disorders and Variations', *American Speech-Language-Hearing Association*, 1993 <https://doi.org/10.1044/policy.RP1993-00208>.

143 'Movement Disorder Society-sponsored Revision of the Unified Parkinson's Disease Rating Scale (MDS-UPDRS): Process, Format, and Clinimetric Testing Plan - Goetz - 2007 - Movement Disorders - Wiley Online Library'
<https://onlinelibrary.wiley.com/doi/full/10.1002/mds.21198> [accessed 25 April 2019].

144 Joseph G. Hentz and others, 'Simplified Conversion Method for Unified Parkinson's Disease Rating Scale Motor Examinations', *Movement Disorders*, 30.14 (2015), 1967–70 <https://doi.org/10.1002/mds.26435>.

145 Pablo Martínez-Martín and others, 'Parkinson's Disease Severity Levels and MDS-Unified Parkinson's Disease Rating Scale', *Parkinsonism & Related Disorders*, 21.1 (2015), 50–54 <https://doi.org/10.1016/j.parkreldis.2014.10.026>.

146 Office of Research & Development, 'Movement Disorder Symptoms Associated with Unified Parkinson's Disease Rating Scale (UPDRS) in Two Manganese (Mn)-Exposed Communities'
<https://cfpub.epa.gov/si/si_public_record_report.cfm?Lab=NHEERL&direntry id=307624> [accessed 25 April 2019].

147 Joseph G. Hentz and others, 'Simplified Conversion Method for Unified Parkinson's Disease Rating Scale Motor Examinations', *Movement Disorders*, 30.14 (2015), 1967–70 <https://doi.org/10.1002/mds.26435>.

148 Office of Research & Development, 'Movement Disorder Symptoms Associated with Unified Parkinson's Disease Rating Scale (UPDRS) in Two Manganese (Mn)-Exposed Communities'
<https://cfpub.epa.gov/si/si_public_record_report.cfm?Lab=NHEERL&direntry id=307624> [accessed 25 April 2019].

149 'Guide.Pdf'

<https://www.alz.washington.edu/NONMEMBER/UDS/DOCS/VER1_2/guid e.pdf> [accessed 25 April 2019].

[150] Margaret M Hoehn, 'Parkinsonism: Onset, Progression, and Mortality', 17.

[151] 'Five Stages of Parkinson's', *Parkinson's Resource Organization* <http://parkinsonsresource.org/news/articles/five-stages-of-parkinsons/> [accessed 25 April 2019].

[152] 'Movement Disorder Society-sponsored Revision of the Unified Parkinson's Disease Rating Scale (MDS-UPDRS): Process, Format, and Clinimetric Testing Plan - Goetz - 2007 - Movement Disorders - Wiley Online Library'.

[153] 'Hoehn and Yahr - Parkinson's Disease Research, Education and Clinical Centers' <https://www.parkinsons.va.gov/resources/HY.asp> [accessed 25 April 2019].

[154] 'Hoehn and Yahr Scale', *Parkinson's Chronicles* <https://www.parkinsonschronicles.com/glossary/hoehn-yahr-scale/> [accessed 25 April 2019].

[155] B. H. Wood and others, 'Incidence and Prediction of Falls in Parkinson's Disease: A Prospective Multidisciplinary Study', *Journal of Neurology, Neurosurgery & Psychiatry*, 72.6 (2002), 721–25 <https://doi.org/10.1136/jnnp.72.6.721>.

[156] 'Activities of Daily Living Questionnaire from Patients' Perspectives in Parkinson's Disease: A Cross-Sectional Study | BMC Neurology | Full Text' <https://bmcneurol.biomedcentral.com/articles/10.1186/s12883-016-0600-9> [accessed 25 April 2019].

[157] 'SCHWAB AND ENGLAND - Parkinson's Disease Research, Education and Clinical Centers' <https://www.parkinsons.va.gov/resources/se.asp> [accessed 25 April 2019].

[158] Claudia Ramaker and others, *Sity Disability Scale [NUDS], Intermediate Scale for Assess-*.

[159] '146_Parkinsons for OT: Module 05' <https://www.atrainceu.com/course-module/2455836-146_parkinsons-for-ot-module-05> [accessed 25 April 2019].

[160] 'Corticobasal Syndrome - Frontotemporal Degeneration', *AFTD* <https://www.theaftd.org/what-is-ftd/corticobasal-syndrome/> [accessed 8 December 2019].

[161] 'Corticobasal Degeneration - Symptoms', *Nhs.Uk*, 2018 <https://www.nhs.uk/conditions/corticobasal-degeneration/symptoms/> [accessed 6 December 2019].

162 'Corticobasal Syndrome - Frontotemporal Degeneration', *AFTD* <https://www.theaftd.org/what-is-ftd/corticobasal-syndrome/> [accessed 6 December 2019].

163 Theodore P. Parthimos and Kleopatra H. Schulpis, 'The Significant Characteristics of Corticobasal Syndrome', *Annals of Research Hospitals*, 3.0 (2019) <http://arh.amegroups.com/article/view/4676> [accessed 11 December 2019].

164 'Dementia with Lewy Bodies Risk Factors', *Alzheimer's Research UK* <https://www.alzheimersresearchuk.org/about-dementia/types-of-dementia/dementia-with-lewy-bodies/risk-factors/> [accessed 24 April 2019].

165 'Research Sheds Light on Risk Factors for DLB | Lewy Body Dementia Association' <https://www.lbda.org/content/research-sheds-light-risk-factors-dlb> [accessed 18 February 2018].

166 Brendon Boot and others, 'Risk Factors for Dementia with Lewy Bodies (S24.005)', *Neurology*, 78.1 Supplement (2012), S24.005-S24.005 <https://n.neurology.org/content/78/1_Supplement/S24.005> [accessed 24 April 2019].

167 'Lewy Body Dementia | Conditions & Treatments | UCSF Medical Center' <https://www.ucsfhealth.org/conditions/lewy_body_dementia/> [accessed 18 February 2018].

168 'Research News | Lewy Body Dementia Association' <https://www.lbda.org/node/1304> [accessed 18 February 2018].

169 'What Are the Risk Factors of Lewy Body Dementia?', *Balance* <https://balance.hcr-manorcare.com/blog-posts/what-are-the-risk-factors-of-lewy-body-dementia/> [accessed 24 April 2019].

170 Genetics Home Reference, 'Dementia with Lewy Bodies', *Genetics Home Reference* <https://ghr.nlm.nih.gov/condition/dementia-with-lewy-bodies> [accessed 24 April 2019].

171 'Lewy Body Dementia: Unrecognized and Misdiagnosed', *Medical News Today* <https://www.medicalnewstoday.com/articles/302230.php> [accessed 24 April 2019].

172 Boot and others.

173 'What Is Dementia with Lewy Bodies?', 12.

174 'Lewy Body Dementia: Information for Patients, Families, and Professionals', 44.

175 'What Causes Lewy Body Dementia?', *National Institute on Aging* <https://www.nia.nih.gov/health/what-causes-lewy-body-dementia> [accessed 24

April 2019].

[176] 'Dementia after Stroke_0.Pdf'
<http://www.stroke.org.uk/sites/default/files/Dementia%20after%20stroke_0.pd
f> [accessed 18 February 2018].

[177] Debby Tsuang and others, 'Association between Lifetime Cigarette
Smoking and Lewy Body Accumulation', *Brain Pathology (Zurich, Switzerland)*, 20.2
(2010), 412–18 <https://doi.org/10.1111/j.1750-3639.2009.00296.x>.

[178] 'Lewy Body Dementia: Information for Patients, Families, and
Professionals | Lewy Body Dementia Association'.

[179] 'Lewy Body Dementia (LBD): Symptoms and Diagnosis', *MedicineNet*
<https://www.medicinenet.com/lewy_body_dementia_dementia_with_lewy_bodi
es/article.htm> [accessed 18 February 2018].

[180] Reference, 'Dementia with Lewy Bodies'.

[181] 'Corticobasal Syndrome', *Memory and Aging Center*
<https://memory.ucsf.edu/dementia/corticobasal-syndrome> [accessed 16
December 2019].

[182] 'Diagnosis | Lewy Body Dementia Association'
<https://www.lbda.org/go/diagnosis-0> [accessed 24 April 2019].

[183] 'Parkinsons_Disease'.

[184] Boot and others.

[185] C.-H. Lin and others, 'Risk of Parkinson's Disease Following
Anxiety Disorders: A Nationwide Population-Based Cohort Study',
European Journal of Neurology, 22.9 (2015), 1280–87
<https://doi.org/10.1111/ene.12740>.

[186] 'Could an Anxiety Disorder Be a Sign of Parkinson's Disease?'
<https://www.hopkinsmedicine.org/health/conditions-and-
diseases/parkinsons-disease/could-an-anxiety-disorder-be-a-sign-of-
parkinsons-disease> [accessed 19 November 2019].

[187] 'Parkinson's Outcomes Project', *Parkinson's Foundation*
<https://www.parkinson.org/research/Parkinsons-Outcomes-Project>
[accessed 19 November 2019].

[188] 'Anxiety', *Parkinson's Foundation*
<https://www.parkinson.org/Understanding-Parkinsons/Symptoms/Non-
Movement-Symptoms/Anxiety> [accessed 19 November 2019].

[189] Samuel M. Goldman, 'Environmental Toxins and Parkinson's Disease',
Annual Review of Pharmacology and Toxicology, 54.1 (2014), 141–64

<https://doi.org/10.1146/annurev-pharmtox-011613-135937>.

[190] 'Research Sheds Light on Risk Factors for DLB | Lewy Body Dementia Association'.

[191] A. G. Schuurman and others, 'Increased Risk of Parkinson's Disease after Depression: A Retrospective Cohort Study', *Neurology*, 58.10 (2002), 1501–4 <https://doi.org/10.1212/wnl.58.10.1501>.

[192] Neuroscience News, 'Increased Risk of Developing Parkinson's Disease in People With Depression', *Neuroscience News*, 2015 <https://neurosciencenews.com/depression-parkinsons-disease-2056/> [accessed 19 November 2019].

[193] Nabila Dahodwala and others, 'Racial Differences in the Diagnosis of Parkinson's Disease', *Movement Disorders : Official Journal of the Movement Disorder Society*, 24.8 (2009), 1200–1205 <https://doi.org/10.1002/mds.22557>.

[194] Stephen K. Van Den Eeden and others, 'Incidence of Parkinson's Disease: Variation by Age, Gender, and Race/Ethnicity', *American Journal of Epidemiology*, 157.11 (2003), 1015–22 <https://doi.org/10.1093/aje/kwg068>.

[195] 'Lewy Body Dementia: Hope Through Research | National Institute of Neurological Disorders and Stroke' <https://www.ninds.nih.gov/Disorders/Patient-Caregiver-Education/Hope-Through-Research/Lewy-Body-Dementia-Hope-Through-Research> [accessed 24 April 2019].

[196] 'Is Dementia Hereditary?', *SeniorAdvisor.Com Blog*, 2016 <https://www.senioradvisor.com/blog/2016/07/is-dementia-hereditary/> [accessed 24 April 2019].

[197] Genetics Home Reference, 'Dementia with Lewy Bodies', *Genetics Home Reference* <https://ghr.nlm.nih.gov/condition/dementia-with-lewy-bodies> [accessed 24 April 2019].

[198] 'SNCA Gene - GeneCards | SYUA Protein | SYUA Antibody' <https://www.genecards.org/cgi-bin/carddisp.pl?gene=SNCA> [accessed 24 April 2019].

[199] Julia M. George, 'The Synucleins', *Genome Biology*, 3.1 (2001), reviews3002.1 <https://doi.org/10.1186/gb-2001-3-1-reviews3002>.

[200] Julia M. George, 'The Synucleins', *Genome Biology*, 3.1 (2001), reviews3002.1 <https://doi.org/10.1186/gb-2001-3-1-reviews3002>.

[201] George, 'The Synucleins'.

[202] Fei Yang and others, 'Socioeconomic Status in Relation to Parkinson's Disease Risk and Mortality', *Medicine*, 95.30 (2016) <https://doi.org/10.1097/MD.0000000000004337>.

[203] M. J. Armstrong and others, 'Roles of Education and IQ in Cognitive Reserve in Parkinson's Disease-Mild Cognitive Impairment', *Dementia and Geriatric Cognitive Disorders Extra*, 2.1 (2012), 343–52 <https://doi.org/10.1159/000341782>.

[204] 'American Academy of Neurology' <https://www.aan.com/> [accessed 24 April 2019].

[205] 'Mayo Clinic Study Finds Occupation And Education Influence Risk For Parkinson's Disease', *ScienceDaily* <https://www.sciencedaily.com/releases/2005/11/051125110756.htm> [accessed 24 April 2019].

[206] Peter T. Nelson and others, 'Association between Male Gender and Cortical Lewy Body Pathology in Large Autopsy Series', *Journal of Neurology*, 257.11 (2010), 1875–81 <https://doi.org/10.1007/s00415-010-5630-4>.

[207] Jessica L. Podcasy and C. Neill Epperson, 'Considering Sex and Gender in Alzheimer Disease and Other Dementias', *Dialogues in Clinical Neuroscience*, 18.4 (2016), 437–46 <https://www.ncbi.nlm.nih.gov/pmc/articles/PMC5286729/> [accessed 9 December 2018].

[208] Siavash Jafari and others, 'Head Injury and Risk of Parkinson Disease: A Systematic Review and Meta-Analysis', *Movement Disorders: Official Journal of the Movement Disorder Society*, 28.9 (2013), 1222–29 <https://doi.org/10.1002/mds.25458>.

[209] Samuel M. Goldman and others, 'Head Injury and Parkinson's Disease Risk in Twins', *Annals of Neurology*, 60.1 (2006), 65–72 <https://doi.org/10.1002/ana.20882>.

[210] Raquel C. Gardner and others, 'Traumatic Brain Injury in Later Life Increases Risk for Parkinson Disease', *Annals of Neurology*, 77.6 (2015), 987–95 <https://doi.org/10.1002/ana.24396>.

[211] 'High Blood Pressure Facts | Cdc.Gov', 2018 <https://www.cdc.gov/bloodpressure/facts.htm> [accessed 24 April 2019].

[212] Neurology Reviews 2016 June;24:41, 'High Blood Pressure Predicts Motor Decline in Parkinson's Disease' <https://www.mdedge.com/neurology/article/109189/movement-disorders/high-blood-pressure-predicts-motor-decline-parkinsons> [accessed 19 November 2019].

213 Jiahao Chen and others, 'Association between Hypertension and the Risk of Parkinson's Disease: A Meta-Analysis of Analytical Studies', *Neuroepidemiology*, 52.3–4 (2019), 181–92 <https://doi.org/10.1159/000496977>.

214 'Monitor Your Blood Pressure', *Www.Heart.Org* <https://www.heart.org/en/health-topics/high-blood-pressure/the-facts-about-high-blood-pressure> [accessed 24 April 2019].

215 Naida L. Graham and others, 'Language Function and Dysfunction in Corticobasal Degeneration', *Neurology*, 61.4 (2003), 493–99 <https://doi.org/10.1212/01.WNL.0000081230.09863.ED>.

216 A. Ascherio and others, 'Prospective Study of Caffeine Consumption and Risk of Parkinson's Disease in Men and Women', *Annals of Neurology*, 50.1 (2001), 56–63.

217 'Coffee Drinking Lowers Risk Of Parkinson's, Type 2 Diabetes, Five Cancers, And More - Harvard Researchers' <https://parkinsonsnewstoday.com/2015/10/02/coffee-drinking-lowers-risk-parkinsons-type-2-diabetes-five-cancers-harvard-researchers/> [accessed 24 April 2019].

218 'Nurses' Health Study |' <https://www.nurseshealthstudy.org/> [accessed 24 April 2019].

219 Ronald B. Postuma and others, 'Caffeine as Symptomatic Treatment for Parkinson Disease (Café-PD): A Randomized Trial', *Neurology*, 89.17 (2017), 1795–1803 <https://doi.org/10.1212/WNL.0000000000004568>.

220 'How Coffee Loves Us Back', *Harvard Gazette*, 2015 <https://news.harvard.edu/gazette/story/2015/09/how-coffee-loves-us-back/> [accessed 24 April 2019].

221 'Genome-Wide Meta-Analysis Identifies Six Novel Loci Associated with Habitual Coffee Consumption | Molecular Psychiatry' <https://www.nature.com/articles/mp2014107> [accessed 24 April 2019].

222 'What's Hot: Coffee Might Not Help with Parkinson's Disease Motor Symptoms', *Parkinson's Foundation*, 2017 <https://parkinson.org/blog/whats-hot/coffee-might-not-help-symptoms> [accessed 24 April 2019].

223 Tanner Caroline M. and others, 'Rotenone, Paraquat, and Parkinson's Disease', *Environmental Health Perspectives*, 119.6 (2011), 866–72 <https://doi.org/10.1289/ehp.1002839>.

224 'CDC | Facts about Paraquat', 2019 <https://emergency.cdc.gov/agent/paraquat/basics/facts.asp> [accessed 24 April 2019].

225 Jesse Kornbluth, 'Poisonous Fallout from the War on Marijuana', *The New York Times*, 19 November 1978, section Archives <https://www.nytimes.com/1978/11/19/archives/poisonous-fallout-from-the-war-on-marijuana-paraquat.html> [accessed 24 April 2019].

226 'DEBATE RAGES AS U.S. PLANS TO SPRAY POT - Chicago Tribune' <https://www.chicagotribune.com/news/ct-xpm-1986-06-01-8602090223-story.html> [accessed 24 April 2019].

227 Katarzyna Kuter and others, 'Increased Reactive Oxygen Species Production in the Brain after Repeated Low-Dose Pesticide Paraquat Exposure in Rats. A Comparison with Peripheral Tissues', *Neurochemical Research*, 35.8 (2010), 1121–30 <https://doi.org/10.1007/s11064-010-0163-x>.

228 'Toxic Influence of Subchronic Paraquat Administration on Dopaminergic Neurons in Rats - ScienceDirect' <https://www.sciencedirect.com/science/article/pii/S0006899307008669?via%3Dihub> [accessed 24 April 2019].

229 'Rotenone - an Overview | ScienceDirect Topics' <https://www.sciencedirect.com/topics/neuroscience/rotenone> [accessed 24 April 2019].

230 Vladimir N. Uversky, 'Neurotoxicant-Induced Animal Models of Parkinson's Disease: Understanding the Role of Rotenone, Maneb and Paraquat in Neurodegeneration', *Cell and Tissue Research*, 318.1 (2004), 225–41 <https://doi.org/10.1007/s00441-004-0937-z>.

231 'Agricultural Health Study (AHS)', *National Institute of Environmental Health Sciences* <https://www.niehs.nih.gov/research/atniehs/labs/epi/studies/ahs/index.cfm> [accessed 24 April 2019].

232 'About the Center | Parkinson's Disease Clinic and Research Center' <https://pdcenter.ucsf.edu/> [accessed 24 April 2019].

233 Genetics Home Reference, 'HCRT Gene', *Genetics Home Reference* <https://ghr.nlm.nih.gov/gene/HCRT> [accessed 24 April 2019].

234 Thomas C. Thannickal, Yuan-Yang Lai, and Jerome M. Siegel, 'Hypocretin (Orexin) Cell Loss in Parkinson's Disease', *Brain*, 130.6 (2007), 1586–95 <https://doi.org/10.1093/brain/awm097>.

235 'REM Sleep Behavior Disorder - Symptoms and Causes - Mayo Clinic' <https://www.mayoclinic.org/diseases-conditions/rem-sleep-behavior-disorder/symptoms-causes/syc-20352920> [accessed 24 April 2019].

236 'Addressing REM Sleep Behavior Disorder in Parkinson's - Neurology Advisor' <https://www.neurologyadvisor.com/topics/neurodegenerative-

diseases/addressing-rem-sleep-behavior-disorder-in-parkinsons/> [accessed 24 April 2019].

237 'BMC, Research in Progress' <https://www.biomedcentral.com/> [accessed 24 April 2019].

238 Yaqian Xu, Jing Yang, and Huifang Shang, *Meta-Analysis of Risk Factors for Parkinson's Disease Dementia*, 2016, V <https://doi.org/10.1186/s40035-016-0058-0>.

239 'Assessment of Neuroinflammation in Patients with Idiopathic Rapid-Eye-Movement Sleep Behaviour Disorder: A Case-Control Study - The Lancet Neurology' <https://www.thelancet.com/journals/laneur/article/PIIS1474-4422(17)30173-4/fulltext> [accessed 24 April 2019].

240 'Restless Sleep May Be an Early Sign of Parkinson's Disease', *EurekAlert!* <https://www.eurekalert.org/pub_releases/2017-12/au-rsm120517.php> [accessed 24 April 2019].

241 Deepak Gupta and Abraham Kuruvilla, 'Vascular Parkinsonism: What Makes It Different?', *Postgraduate Medical Journal*, 87.1034 (2011), 829–36 <https://doi.org/10.1136/postgradmedj-2011-130051>.

242 'Vascular (Multi-Infarct) Parkinsonism | Healthcare | Baylor College of Medicine | Houston, Texas' <https://www.bcm.edu/healthcare/care-centers/parkinsons/conditions/vascular-parkinsonism> [accessed 24 April 2019].

243 'Wiley: Poor Diet May Increase Risk of Parkinson's Disease' <https://www.wiley.com/WileyCDA/PressRelease/pressReleaseId-112174.html> [accessed 24 April 2019].

244 'Diagnosis and Management of Dementia with Lewy Bodies | Neurology' <https://n.neurology.org/content/89/1/88> [accessed 24 April 2019].

245 Betsy Simmons Hannibal and Attorney, 'How to Write a Living Will', *Www.Nolo.Com* <https://www.nolo.com/legal-encyclopedia/how-write-living-will.html> [accessed 21 November 2019].

246 'Power of Attorney' <https://www.americanbar.org/groups/real_property_trust_estate/resources/estate_planning/power_of_attorney/> [accessed 22 November 2019].

247 'Treatment and Management of Lewy Body Dementia', *National Institute on Aging* <https://www.nia.nih.gov/health/treatment-and-management-lewy-body-dementia> [accessed 24 April 2019].

www.ingramcontent.com/pod-product-compliance
Lightning Source LLC
Chambersburg PA
CBHW030622220526
45463CB00004B/1378